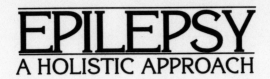

EPILEPSY
A HOLISTIC APPROACH

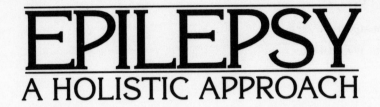

EPILEPSY

A HOLISTIC APPROACH

A simple guide on how to help
your epilepsy through the use of
alternative and complementary medicine

CAROLINE THOMAS

Published in 1993
by Images Publishing (Malvern) Ltd,
13 Old Street,
Upton-upon-Severn,
Worcs. WR8 0HN.

in conjunction with
Caroline Thomas

British Library Cataloguing in Publication Data

A catalogue record for this book is available from the British Library

ISBN 1 897817 09 6

Designed and Produced by Images Publishing (Malvern) Ltd.
Printed & Bound in Great Britain.

Contents

Introduction

Epilepsy can be very distressing both for the individual with the condition and for the friends and family. Often the cause is not clear and this can make it hard to treat. For many people, once their medication is stabilised they have no more fits and are quite happy. Unfortunately, for many others this is not the case.

The best description that I have come across describing the emotional effect of epilepsy was written by Mayer and Gutjahr and says:

> With each new adaptation or change of medication resulting in a seizure free period comes the hope of being completely seizure free until the next attack destroys these hopes . . . The patient experiences in his illness and social situation a feeling of helplessness and comes against an apparently unbreakable social chain that forces on him a feeling of dependence.

This book is for those who feel that more can be done to control their epilepsy but are not really sure what to do and where to go to for advice. There are legal restrictions against treating epilepsy to protect people from wonder cures that could do more damage than good. Although this form of protection offered to patients is welcome, it also means that alternative practitioners may sometimes find that they are not allowed to give all the help they could. However, many practitioners have treated epileptic patients for various other problems and found that the epilepsy improved as well. Various practitioners have also found that even if the treatment has not reduced the number of fits, it has managed to reduce the severity of them, or just make the patient's life easier to handle.

The main aim of most doctors, when it comes to treating epilepsy, seems to be to reduce the number of fits that occur. However, many patients that I have met are more concerned about the quality of life.

It is no use having no fits if the side effects of the drugs that you are taking mean that you sleep half the day and are dopey the other half. Unfortunately, if your doctor treats you in any other way he can get into trouble, or at least be accused of not treating the patient properly.

This is why I feel there is a need to produce a book on self-help, a book to collate all the existing information on the topic and pass it onto the people who really need it – those suffering from epilepsy.

This book is divided into two main parts. The first part (chapters 1 to 7) looks at possible causes of the fits and ways to eliminate them. The second part looks at methods that have been shown to help patients when no cause has been found. To make full use of this book, the first part should be read and considered, and then the chapters in the second part can be read in any order you wish. At the back is a list of names and addresses and other information that you may find useful.

I have included many case studies throughout the book, in most cases the names are changed to protect anonymity. I also use the word *fit*, which can be considered a vague term, to cover *petit mal*, *grand mal* and any other types of attacks, unless a more specific term is required in the circumstances.

Unfortunately, with most forms of alternative medicine it is difficult to do the sort of tests to prove whether the treatment works or not as required by our drug companies, because the treatment is much more individual. However, many of the older drugs on the market were produced before the strict regulations were brought in and are still used. I have met and heard of many people who are certain that a specific method worked for them. Added to this, it is extremely unlikely that there will be any side effects from alternative treatments.

It is also important to remember that epilepsy is often considered a sign of intelligence and many famous people, including St Paul, Mohammed, Julius Caesar, Napoleon and Swedenborg, were all epileptic and they still managed to lead productive lives. There are a variety of more recent epileptics as well, although unfortunately they tend to keep it quiet.

Causes

Fits can be caused by a variety of factors, and in well over half of the cases the cause remains unknown. Some people believe that perhaps we all have epileptic tendencies and, given the correct conditions, will all have convulsions. A very high proportion of people will have at least one convulsion in their life, usually when ill and in early childhood. If the reasons are unknown and the fits continue then the patient is considered to be epileptic. Unfortunately there are many causes of fits that may not be considered, and so drugs are given to repress the symptoms rather than getting to the root of the problem. Allergies are the most obvious example. Just by bearing this in mind it may be possible to find a trigger for your epilepsy, perhaps something you have eaten, somewhere you have been, someone you have been with or the time of day. Since stress plays a major part in epilepsy, something that concerns you may also affect the condition.

Many of the possible causes cannot be treated. It is said that in a noticeable amount of cases of epilepsy there was a problem birth perhaps leading to neck or head injuries, there are many cases where parents or grandparents drank excessively and where there was a family history of neurosis. Electroconvulsant treatment can also initiate epilepsy. There are also connections with various immunisations, especially measles. There are various bodily imbalances that are considered to affect epilepsy and these will be discussed in future chapters.

Simple Treatment

It is important to have the necessary tests to investigate whether the fits have a physical cause and whether there is the possibility of the patient suffering from brain damage or a tumour. Although this is not very likely, without you already knowing about it, it is essential that it is caught early if there should be.

The first recommendations given to epileptics are those given to most people for a healthy life, to try and make your life as stable as possible. Obviously this is not always easy but even regular meals and regular sleeping hours can make a lot of difference. Take regular, but not excessive exercise, eat properly and keep stress to a minimum. Sometimes alcohol can trigger attacks, but if you are sure that this is not a problem in your case then drinking can be allowed, as long as it is not in excess. Do bear in mind, though, that alcohol can react with any anticonvulsants that you may be on, although your doctor should have told you about this. Smoking is not recommended.

The body, by nature, tries to heal itself and, given a stable and nutritional background, it can strengthen its resources to do this. If you do change your diet and lifestyle do it slowly, don't change everything all at once. In sensitive cases, which epileptics often are, sudden changes can shake your body up considerably causing short term problems, and this may well increase the chances of having a fit. In addition to this, it is possible that boredom or stress will set in if too much effort is needed by starting many things at once. Besides, if everything is tried at once it will be very hard to know what is actually having an effect.

PART I

Causes and Ways to Avoid Them

Chapter 1 - Allergies

Introduction

Allergies can be responsible for epileptic fits. If your fits are infrequent then it may be easy to tell if there is anything that may have triggered them off; if they are frequent it is not so easy. Allergies which lead to fits tend to be chemical based, but this is not necessarily so. If you are the sort of person who suffers from hay fever, skin rashes and other allergic symptoms, then it is more likely that your epilepsy is also allergy based. Even if your fits seem to be stress based there still could be an allergic element. There are two reasons for this: firstly there are chemical changes that occur in the body when under stress that make you more susceptible to allergies; secondly you may eat differently - and extra sweets and chocolate that are very commonly eaten when under stress are more likely to lead to fits. There are certain chemicals that should be particularly avoided by epileptics.

Every individual has their own specific organs where the allergic reaction is likely to occur. In some cases this can be the brain, and this may lead to fits. Allergic reactions in the brain can lead to a varied range of behavioural changes.

Allergies tend to run in the family, so if both parents suffer from allergies it is very likely that the children will also; if one parent suffers from allergies, some of the children may also. However, the actual substances to which the individual reacts, may be completely different from one person to the next, as may the reactions it brings.

There has been a massive increase in the number of allergic people during the last century as there has been great increase in the adulteration of food and the amount of chemicals used. It is hard to tell if there are more epileptics now than there were before, partly because, especially in the past, people would not admit to it. Some people say that allergies are all in the mind and may be due to some emotional connection in the past. Whilst this is definitely the case sometimes, it is not usually so.

There are a wide variety of other allergic symptoms that can arise, and if you find that you are suffering from a few of those symptoms shown in the table below, especially in the nervous system section, you are quite probably suffering from allergies of some sort. Therefore it is quite possible that your epilepsy is an allergic reaction as well.

Area	Symptoms
Central Nervous System	Extreme exhaustion Headaches Migraines Sleep disorders and nightmares Snoring Grinding of teeth Difficulties in reading and comprehension Deteriorating writing Clumsiness Facial tics Trembling Tingling or pins and needles Restlessness Fidgety legs Loss of balance Giddiness Extreme weakness Lack of energy Epilepsy
Chest	Recurrent bronchitis and asthma A choking, suffocating feeling

Digestive System	Cravings for some foods
	Loss of appetite
	Bingeing
	Anorexia Nervosa
	Bulimia
	Diarrhoea
	Stomach pains
	Stomach and mouth ulcers
	Weight problems
	Bilious attacks
	Wind
	Bloated stomach
	Swollen abdominal glands – Mesenteric adenitis
	Irritable bowel syndrome
	Piles
	Regular constipation
	Abnormal thirst
	Colitis
	Crohn's disease
Ears	Oversensitivity to noise
	Deafness
	Glue ear
Eyes	Pain when looking at bright lights
	Dislike of bright lights
	Fluctuations of vision
	Bags under the eyes
	Shadows under the eyes
	Dry eyes
	Feeling of grit in the eyes
Genito-Urinary System	Persistent cystitis
	Bed wetting
	Loss of sexual desire
	Impotence
	Prostatis
	Recurrent thrush
	Pre-menstrual tension
	Heavy periods

Hair	Greasy hair
	Dry hair
	Premature greying
	Premature baldness
	Dandruff
Heart	Fast or slow pulse
	Coronary thrombosis
Joints	Painful and aching joints
	Audible clicking in the joints
	Arthritis
Mind	Violent mood swings
	Aggression
	Panic attacks
	Lack of concentration
	Incoherence
	Bad memory
	Delusions
	Hallucinations
	Alcohol and drug addiction
Mouth	Bad breath
	Bad taste
	Loss of taste
	Sore tongue
	Bleeding gums
	Dry and cracked lips
	Dry tongue and mouth
	Mouth ulcers
Nails	Nail biting
Nose	Snuffly nose
	Catarrh
	Constantly runny nose
	Acute sense of smell
	No sense of smell

Skin	Acne, eczema and other rashes
	Weals
	Hypersensitivity to touch
	Dry flaking skin
	Greasy skin
	Excessive sweating
	Excessive bruising
Throat	Recurrent sore throats
	Continuous dry cough
Other	Bodily secretions
	Inexplicable fevers
	Feelings of extreme heat or cold
	Premature ageing
	Breast pains
	Weight fluctuations

E numbers to be avoided

Fits can be initiated by certain foods and food additives. It may be worth trying to avoid the following additives to see if this makes any difference.

E210 – Benzoic acid – This occurs naturally in many fruits and vegetables and is also chemically produced as a food additive. The most likely effects that benzoic acid will have is asthma and urticaria (nettle rash). However, it may also cause digestive upsets and may be responsible for some neurological disorders. It is also thought to react with sodium bisulphite (E222) and to produce hyperactivity in some children. The natural form of additives are often less likely to cause problems than the chemical version.

E141 – Copper complexes of chlorophyll and of chlorophyllins
E141(i) – Copper complexes of chlorophyll
E141(ii) – Copper complexes of chlorophyll
E173 – Aluminium
E519 – Cupric sulphate

E541 – Sodium aluminium phosphate acidic (SAP)

E541 – Sodium aluminium phosphate basic

E554 – Aluminium sodium silicate (sodium aluminsilicate)

E556 – Aluminium calcium silicate

E559 – Aluminium silicate – Excess aluminium and copper is known to effect epilepsy, therefore it is a good idea to avoid these when possible. In cases where the cause could be hereditary it is possibly a good idea for brothers, sisters and children to avoid it as well, as a precaution, because sometimes the damage can be irreparable. Aluminium may be responsible for Parkinson type diseases and Alzheimer's disease (senile dementia) too. Some people believe that high aluminium intakes may be harmful to patients with bone disease or kidney impairment.

E924 – Potassium bromate – Potassium bromate is used in producing flour and beer. If used in excess quantities it can lead to nausea, vomiting, diarrhoea and convulsions, but it shouldn't have any effects if taken in normal quantities.

Alcohol

Between 4% and 20% of alcoholics are thought to have convulsive seizures. Different figures have been found in different studies. However it does show that excess alcohol can lead to convulsions. Convulsions are also common after alcohol withdrawal, but this wears off.

Having said this, in one test about 80% of alcohol users find no association between convulsions and alcohol, and only 5% found a frequent association. Basically, it is worth investigating whether your fits (convulsions or not) seem to be related to alcohol. One way to do this may be to make a chart of when and how much you drink and when and how severe are the fits. If there seems to be a correlation, cut out alcohol for a few weeks and see if the pattern changes.

Other Foods to Avoid

Foods and drinks that are stimulants and irritants should be avoided, these include such things as coffee, sugar, excess salt, chocolate, cola, animal protein and spices. This is because they suddenly change the metabolism of your body and this can trigger off fits. As before, it is probably a good idea to remove these from your diet for a few weeks. If you find that there is no improvement then you can revert to taking them again. If you buy decaffeinated coffee, be careful to buy one that is processed without too many chemicals.

General Procedures

If you think that your problem might be allergy-based it is worth keeping a note of when you have your fits and what may have triggered them. You will probably find some pattern that helps you find the root of your problem. There are various tests for finding your allergies and, although none of them are considered completely reliable, they can often help. Eliminating the things that they consider you may be allergic to can make life much easier and perhaps makes it easier for you to decide if there is anything else that may be affecting you. One, fairly easy method of testing an allergic reaction is by measuring the pulse. When you consume something that you are allergic to, your pulse will usually start racing. Although this is not completely reliable, it is something that with a little bit of practise can be very helpful in getting to the root of allergic reactions.

Other methods exist, such as putting people on a fast for a few days or a diet of foods that very seldom cause allergies (such as pears and lamb), and then slowly bringing in more foods until the reactions start again. Obviously this procedure is rather impractical if you are having fits every few months, but if they're frequent then it may be helpful. If you are having fits every few months you will probably find that other symptoms, maybe that you have never connected, will clear up too, or you will just feel generally better. It is very important to eliminate everything from your diet that you know does cause you problems. It also may be a good idea to take a note of everything you have eaten just before each fit as well as the chemicals that you have been involved with. This may give some idea.

In the case of women, if your fits occur at the same stage during your menstrual cycle, check whether you eat a lot of sweets (which is the usual thing) or anything else at this time. Try cutting them out and seeing if this makes any difference, and look at the low blood sugar chapter.

When removing a substance to which you are allergic, you may find that for a couple of days you feel worse. This is due to your body adjusting to the change and is trying to remove all poisons from the body. This shouldn't last for long, and afterwards you should start feeling noticeably better, which in turn should encourage you to avoid the substance further.

There are many good books on allergies, and you can probably pick one up at your library. There are also people who specialise in sorting out your allergies and some relevant associations. For more information on these see the Appendix.

There are various vitamins and minerals that help strengthen the immune system and clear the body of toxins. Herbs are also available. For more information on these, see the relevant chapters, and the chapter on Detoxification.

Other Available Tests

There are a variety of tests that are available for testing allergies. The IgE test is a blood test that measures the level of one of the proteins that shows antibody activity. If this is high then you are susceptible to allergies. A RAST test is similar to the IgE test but measures the response to a specific food. Unfortunately most people who have a tendency to allergies will know this, which may make the IgE test something of a waste of time. The use of the RAST test requires some idea of what the individual is allergic to. Also available on the NHS are skin prick and patch tests that place the substance direct on the skin to see whether there is any reaction.

Not available on the NHS, however, is the hair test. Some people say this is of no use at all, but some people say it is wonderful. Since

22

only a small sample of hair is required, which should be taken from the nape of the neck, it is possibly the easiest test for the patient. The sample of hair is usually sent in by post. It will then be tested against a variety of common allergens and a list of anything you may be allergic to will be sent to you. Although not free, this test is fairly cheap, especially if you shop around. A few addresses will be found in the Appendix.

Another test is the Vega test. It is completely painless and takes the form of a simple electric circuit where both the patient being tested and the substance which may cause allergy are connected; a little dial will show how the body reacts to it. This test is also used to measure vitamin and mineral deficiency and is sometimes found in health food shops. Addresses for this can be found in the Appendix.

Unfortunately, although these tests can help considerably, the only reliable way of testing for allergies is to remove the substance completely and see what happens. It is important that you get to know exactly what ingredients you are eating. This can sometimes be very difficult, but you should persevere.

Other Treatment

When you have found out what is the cause of your allergy, there are two main options available to you. First of all you can simply avoid the substance that causes the problem. This is often inconvenient or frustrating but, if possible, should be tried. If this cannot be done then your doctor can provide desensitisation drops that will help, and after a few sessions may eliminate the problem completely.

Case Study

Mary was diagnosed as epileptic at the age of eight. She was given various drugs, many of which had unacceptable side effects, but finally settled on Epilim and Epanutin that didn't seem to disagree with her. In adulthood the fits were happening about once a month. That was less often than when she was younger, but the efficiency of the drugs was always in doubt by her family. At the age of 23 she decided to come off the anticonvulsants and in the seven years since then has only had two fits. The first one occurred when she had a cold and took some expectorant, which has been known occasionally to initiate fits in susceptible people. The second occasion happened when she was also unwell and the bedroom in which she was sleeping was being painted. She also suffers from various other allergies such as hay fever and an allergy to chocolate, so it seems likely that both those cases were caused by allergic reactions.

Chapter 2 – Vitamins and Minerals

Introduction

Many people have found that having the correct amounts of vitamins and minerals can have an amazing effect on their epilepsy and on their general well-being. Even if you are having the recommended daily intake of vitamins and minerals, it is possible that your body needs more because everybody's requirements are slightly different. If you are under stress, some vitamins and minerals including vitamins B and C are used up much more. Additionally, if you sweat a great deal, many of the vitamins and minerals will be lost, so it is particularly important to have an adequate intake during the summer. It is always best, if possible, to get your necessary nutrients from a healthy diet rather than supplements. This is not always easy, especially as much of the food available now has been processed to a degree where much of the goodness has been lost from it. Many of the anticonvulsants can deplete nutrient levels, which in turn can possibly cause fits. Therefore it is essential to keep these nutrient levels up.

I have listed below, the various nutrients that can affect epilepsy, along with other symptoms that may arise, and the recommended intakes. These are often more than the standard recommended daily intake, and it is quite possible that you only need some of these nutrients. A good quality multi vitamin and mineral pill may well provide you with many of these nutrients. The effect of an increase in some of the vitamins will be almost instantaneous. However, an increase in some of the minerals can take as long as a few months to have a noticeable effect. I would suggest that you don't suddenly go out and buy loads of different vitamins and minerals and start taking them all at once, because this may shake up your body and increase the number of fits for a little while, until you have adjusted to the new intake. If you are taking more than one type of supplement, leave a week between starting the first type and then starting the second type, longer if you feel this is necessary. If your fits are infrequent it may be practical to leave a few months between taking the different supplements, so that you can see if there is any change. It may be also sensible to increase the dosage slowly, so if the recommended dosage is three a day, take one a day for a few days, then go onto two a day and then three a day. Of course, this way it is also easier to tell which supplements have an effect. However, in certain circumstances it is recommended that a combination is needed; in these cases the complete combination should be taken.

You may feel that it would be sensible to visit a nutritional therapist who will be experienced in analysing the nutritional requirements of individuals. It is possible to get tests done that will give you some indication of where you are lacking in vitamins and minerals. See the names and addresses section in the Appendix for this. Your local health food shop probably will have a better choice and higher quality supplements than your chemist. In addition to this, they should be able to give you any advice that you need. If you have difficulty getting hold of any of the pills, look at the name and address section in the Appendix.

Low blood sugar is also a possible nutritional problem, and in many cases this can be easily controlled (see Chapter 6). The contents of the previous chapter on allergies also should be borne in mind when using dietary methods for treatment.

The units in which vitamins and minerals are measured can sometimes be a bit complicated since they can vary. However, careful reading of the jar should always make this easier. To decide on what vitamins and minerals to take, read through the following list and work out which ones are most suitable to your health problems.

Vitamins

A

The recommended intake of vitamin A for epileptics is the same as that for other people: 750µg, which is 2,500 International Units (IU).

Do not take more than double this amount without medical supervision, also, do not take vitamin A supplements if you are pregnant. Deficiencies lead to eye problems, repeated infections and poor skin and hair quality. Vegans will be particularly at risk as will those who take drugs, drink too much alcohol or coffee or smoke. Good sources of vitamin A are fish, liver, egg yolk, cream and green leafy or yellow vegetables.

B COMPLEX

When taking vitamin B it is usually better to take a B complex rather than just B_6 or B_{12} or any other individual member. This is because they work together and a balance of the parts is important.

If you feel stressed then you will probably require quite a high intake of a B Complex. This can cause a vicious circle since a lack of B vitamins can make you feel tense and feeling tense can use up a lot of B vitamins. If you feel that this may be part of your problem make sure that you read the chapter on low blood sugar. In this case it is often necessary to have a high intake for a short time until you find that you are generally fairly relaxed, and then cut down the dosage. A daily dosage of 100-200mg may be required, this is often best split into doses 2 or 3 times a day. Find a jar of supplements that has this sort of volume on its recommended intake, rather than taking large quantities of pills designed to be taken in smaller quantities. The best way of judging if you are having too much vitamin B is the colour of your urine. Excess of certain B vitamins will cause it to be very yellow. This is the only side effect and does no damage, but if you find that your urine is still yellow even when you are due to take your next pill, then you are probably having too much and should cut down.

Other symptoms of inadequate vitamin B are tiredness, premenstrual syndrome, lack of appetite, lack of concentration and eye problems. B complex deficiencies are particularly common in those who smoke, drink alcohol, who don't eat much meat and who are on the contraceptive pill.

27

B_6 has known properties as an anticonvulsant, and additional amounts of this may be taken. However, it is known that more than 200mg a day of B_6 taken regularly for over a year can cause problems. That sort of intake is rather excessive and should not be necessary, except, perhaps, as a short term measure. B_6 can also be destroyed by some of the anticonvulsants.

Often folic acid, which is another member of the B complex, is recommended by the doctors since this is destroyed by many anticonvulsants. It sometimes gives a reduction in fit frequency and it often gives an improvement in peripheral symptoms such as mental state, mood, intellectual speed, alertness, concentration, self confidence, independence and sociability. However, since it is often given anyway, many epileptics will already be having sufficient amounts. If you are taking a good B complex, this is probably not necessary. However, if you are pregnant and not taking any B supplements it is probably a very good idea to have some extra folic acid or brewer's yeast. This is one of the most important nutrients used to treat the condition.

B_{12} is also sometimes given. A deficiency of B_{12} can lead to tiredness, loss of appetite, poor memory, paranoia, pernicious anaemia and a smooth sore tongue.

The best source of the B vitamins are brewer's yeast, yeast extract, offal, wheat and rice.

C

Vitamin C is easily destroyed during cooking. Much of our processed food is lacking in vitamin C. If you are under stress, much of the body's vitamin C will be destroyed, so it is important to have an adequate amount. Amongst many other things, vitamin C helps produce brain and nerve substances, so it is important to have enough. It is also important for the gums, which can be affected by some of the anticonvulsants. Those under stress, those who smoke, diabetics and those who are on the contraceptive pill should have more than the recommended intake.

The recommended daily intake is about 60mg but anything up to

1000mg (1g) is sometimes required. More than 3g of vitamin C on a regular basis may cause problems, so keep well below this amount.

The most obvious signs of a deficiency of vitamin C are colds and bleeding gums; lethargy and irritability can also occur. The best sources of vitamin C are rosehips, citrus fruits, blackcurrants, cabbage, Brussels sprouts, tomatoes and potatoes. As it is often destroyed by boiling, where possible these foods should be taken raw or only lightly cooked.

D

Vitamin D is depleted by the intake of anticonvulsants. Supplements of this should not exceed 10μg. The recommended daily intake in most countries is 2.5μg, although in some countries it is as much as 10μg. If you spend a reasonable length of time in the sun it is probably not necessary to have supplements. However, in the winter, or if you don't like the sun, supplements may be necessary. Deficiency is more common in vegetarians and those of Asian descent (due to the diet and skin type). Deficiency symptoms are muscular spasms and weakness, pain in the bones, and brittle bones. The best sources of vitamin D are sunlight, halibut and cod liver oil, oily fish, tuna, eggs, butter and milk.

E

Vitamin E is another vitamin that is destroyed by cooking. The recommended daily intake is at least 30mg. Deficiency will result in apathy, irritability and lack of concentration. It reduces the oxygen needs of the muscles which means that it should help if your problem is affected by a lack of oxygen to the brain, for example, if you have a chest problem. A common intake for treatment can be 500IU or more. Deficiency can be caused by contraceptive pills and air pollution. The best sources of vitamin E are vegetable and fish oils, wheatgerm, leafy vegetables, egg yolk, legumes, lettuce, peanuts and wholewheat flour.

Minerals

CALCIUM

Calcium is used during the treatment of epilepsy, due to its sedative effects. It also affects the absorption of magnesium, so it is often a good idea to take the two together. It is possible to get pills containing a combination of calcium and magnesium. Extra calcium is given to those who have bone problems, allergy problems, depression, anxiety, menstrual pains and muscle and joint pains. If you are on the contraceptive pill, pregnant or breast feeding, extra calcium may be needed. The recommended intake of calcium is 500-1500mg. The best sources of calcium are cheese, fish, nuts, root vegetables and eggs.

CHROMIUM

Chromium is important for blood sugar control. It stimulates the production of essential nerve substances. Deficiency can result in nervousness. Chromium is sometimes used in the treatment of low blood sugar. Those most likely to be at risk from chromium deficiency are the elderly, those who drink alcohol, those who are slimming or pregnant and those with a high intake of refined foods. There is no recommended daily intake but a safe and adequate range is given as 50-200µg. The best sources of chromium are yeast, liver, cheese, fruit juices, wholewheat and wheatgerm.

GERMANIUM

This mineral induces more oxygen into the blood stream, and again, may be particularly useful if you have chest problems. The recommended daily intake is about 200mg.

MAGNESIUM

Convulsions are a known effect of a magnesium deficiency, as are weakness and tiredness, nervousness, muscle cramps, tremors and

30

twitching, especially around the eyes. The recommended daily intake is about 400mg. More may be needed if you suffer from allergies, pre-menstrual syndrome or menstrual cramps, or are suffering from morning sickness or hypoglycemia (low blood sugar), or if on the contraceptive pill or antibiotics. More magnesium is needed for those who have a high intake of fluoride – this can occur in areas with flouridated water and in those who drink a lot of tea. The suggested supplementation of magnesium is 500-1000mg. Magnesium tablets should be taken in conjunction with calcium. There are tablets available which combine the two. The most absorbable form of magnesium is magnesium chloride and this is best taken on an empty stomach, at least half an hour before eating. This is one of the most important nutrients used to treat epilepsy. The best sources of magnesium are soya beans, nuts, brown rice, fish and lentils.

MANGANESE

This can be used in the treatment of epilepsy. One of the functions of manganese is to maintain a healthy nervous system. The recommended daily intake is between 2.5mg and 5mg, but up to half this intake can be provided by tea drinking. The best source of manganese are soya beans, nuts and brewer's yeast.

SELENIUM

Selenium is very useful in detoxifying the body. However, it can be fatal if taken in excess, the maximum daily dose is 200µg and no more than this should be taken. It is known to help in cancer and angina cases as well as arthritis and high blood pressure. Its most common natural sources are organ meats, fish and shellfish.

ZINC

The quantity of zinc is greatly reduced by the refining and processing of food. It is also reduced by anticonvulsants, smoking, alcohol and the contraceptive pill. The recommended daily intake is about 12mg although at least 50mg is often recommended. It is thought that intakes of over 150mg per day may occasionally have side effects. Zinc is used to treat mild mental conditions and to supplement schizophrenics. The most obvious sign of deficiency is white spots on finger nails, eczema of face and hands, acne, mental apathy and loss of sense of taste and smell. The best sources of zinc are oysters, meat, pumpkin seeds, cheese and eggs.

Amino Acids

DIMETHYL-GLYCINE (DMG)

DMG is also known as B15. It is an amino acid that has been used to treat epilepsy. It helps to stimulate your immune system. Therefore, a lack of this can mean that you keep getting infections. It also helps increase the amount of oxygen to the brain, so may be particularly helpful if you have chest problems. Supplements of about 90mg twice a day can have a noticeable effect.

TAURINE

Taurine is one of the lesser known amino acids, but is known to have an effect in the treatment of epilepsy. The recommended daily dosage of this is 1-3g. Taurine deficiency can lead to facial twitches too. The balance of amino acids can be very disturbed in epileptics and additional taurine can help balance this and lead to improved brain function. It also helps balance the zinc/copper ratio that helps because often zinc is low and copper high in epileptics. Adequate zinc is important to the correct processing of taurine. This is one of the most important nutrients used to treat the condition. Taurine is produced in the body and is found in animal proteins.

TYROSINE

Tyrosine is another amino acid that is sometimes used to treat epilepsy. A shortage of this may lead to pale hair and skin. The recommended dosage of this is 500mg three times a day and this should lead to improved brain function.

Other nutrients

LECITHIN

One of the functions of lecithin is as a part of the myelin sheath that is an insulator around the nerves. Lecithin is used to reduce high blood pressure, reduce blood cholesterol levels and reduce blood fat levels. The recommended intake for treatment is 4 capsules three times per day, or in granular form in drinks or on food. The best sources of lecithin are wheat, soya beans and peanuts.

ADRENAL EXTRACT

The adrenal gland produces, amongst other things, an anti-stress hormone. Therefore, adrenal extract can have a stabilising effect on the mental state.

DIGESTIVE ENZYMES

It is possible that the number of fits is increased by an inefficient digestive system since this means the necessary nutrients will not be absorbed completely from the food eaten. In this case extra digestive enzymes will help this absorption.

EFA (ESSENTIAL FATTY ACIDS)

There is still a great deal to be learnt about essential fatty acids. The most common symptom of a deficiency of these is dermatitis. However, it has sometimes been found to be helpful in the treatment of epilepsy, the recommended supplement being four capsules three times a day.

KELP

This is a form of seaweed and is an excellent source of minerals. Five tablets of kelp a day can have some effect.

PANCREATIC ENZYMES

Convulsions can be affected by glandular imbalances in the pancreas. Therefore some pancreatic enzymes can help stabilise this. It can also help blood sugar levels.

PITUITARY EXTRACT

The pituitary glands have many functions, including stimulating other glands. Therefore pituitary extract can help the body function correctly in a variety of ways.

PROTEOLYTIC ENZYMES

These help the digestion and hence the production of various nutrients including amino acids. Extra proteolytic enzymes can help epilepsy by increasing the body's production of the nutrients that will help the condition. These should be taken between meals.

RAW THYMUS CONCENTRATE

The thymus is a gland whose main aim is the development of the immune system and resistance to infection. Therefore raw thymus concentrate can help if you tend to get many infections. It also helps to improve brain function.

THYROID EXTRACT

The thyroid gland helps in the processing of protein and therefore the production of amino acids. Amino acids are very helpful in the treatment of epilepsy. Thyroid extract can increase the production of amino acids and it can also help improve brain function. Additional thyroid extract may be particularly important if you eat large quantities of peanuts or cabbage since these tend to reduce the normal production of thyroid.

Case Studies

Michael was in his thirties and having frequent petit mal attacks. His general diet was improved and he took additional B complex, magnesium, multi mineral and taurine. After this he was much improved. In time his supplements lapsed and the attacks returned. However as soon as the regime was restored he improved again.

Susan had suffered from grand mal from the age of 18 months until she was in her teens. From then until she was 32 she was seizure and medication free. At 32 the seizures returned. There were some obvious problems with her digestive system. She was found to be gluten sensitive, and this caused drops in the blood sugar level and also reduced the absorption of nutrients. By excluding gluten and giving supplements of B complex and magnesium along with vitamins, multi minerals, calcium and digestive enzymes, she has been seizure free for 13 years.

David was 22 and had a long history of generalised epileptic seizures. When he was given supplements of 90mg of dimethyl glycine (DMG) twice daily the seizures were reduced from 16 to 3 a week. When the DMG was withdrawn the seizures returned to their previous level.

John was 41 and had had a history of epilepsy although it had recently got much worse. He was having about three petit mals a day and some grand mals. He had a history of chest problems so it was thought that maybe dimethyl glycine would help, since there was probably a reduced flow of oxygen to the brain. He was given two 125mg tablets of DMG a day and an improvement was noticed almost immediately. He has had no grand mals since and only a few petit mals, usually when he is feeling unwell generally.

Chapter 3 – Hormones

Introduction

A very high proportion of women find that their fits take place at period time. Many of the others find that they take place at ovulation time (about two weeks before the period starts). They often find that the fits stop if they go on the contraceptive pill or if they get pregnant or are breast feeding.

With men it is obviously harder to measure whether fits have a hormonal link. However, many men believe that they do have a hormonal cycle, although the length of this can vary considerably, and if you have fits every one to two months this is quite possibly part of the problem.

Therefore, with women, your doctor may suggest that you go on the pill or perhaps have some hormone treatment. While this is possibly worth considering, alternative medicine believes that it is not getting to the root of the problem. There must be a reason for the hormones not to be correctly balanced in the first place. The most likely cause for this is that you are suffering from a low blood sugar problem, and more on this can be seen in Chapter 6. In mild cases you may find that some very simple changes to your lifestyle may solve the problem; in other cases these changes may be more severe.

Other treatments that may help this are any natural treatments used for pre-menstrual syndrome (PMS), which can cover many symptoms, including fits. Some of these are covered in other areas of this book. If you believe that this is your problem, it is worth keeping a note of all your other symptoms as they occur and perhaps looking under the vitamin and mineral chapter too. You may lack in certain vitamins and minerals at period time as there are substantial changes in the body metabolism. However, I would strongly recommend reading the chapter on low blood sugar and experimenting with this first. There are many treatments for pre-menstrual syndrome on the shelves of health food shops, and it may well be worth trying them to see if you can come up with something that works for you. It is also important to avoid stress as much as possible and to take enough exercise.

Evening primrose oil is recommended for the treatment of PMS. Unfortunately those with temporal lobe epilepsy are advised against evening primrose oil because it can cause fits.

Other recommended vitamins and minerals are listed below. Further information on these can be seen in the chapter on vitamins and minerals

- Vitamin A
- Vitamin B Complex
- Vitamin C
- Calcium
- Vitamin E
- EPA – (eicosapentaenoic acid)
- Magnesium
- Raw adrenal tablets
- Raw pituitary tablets
- Zinc

There are a variety of books available on this topic and there are books and addresses on this topic in Appendix 2.

Chapter 4 – Relaxation

Introduction

The ability to relax is essential for the successful treatment of epilepsy and many other conditions. However, it is possibly more important in the treatment of epilepsy, since epilepsy can be very stress based and stress causing.

There are a great variety of ways to relax, and to a certain extent it depends on the individual as to what is best and most practical. There are a variety of treatments in other chapters of this book that will definitely help, but there are also a variety of other methods. It is also essential to remove any stress causing factors that you can, if only temporarily while you try to sort yourself out in other ways.

The most important thing is to have a little while, ideally every day, to do what you want and when you are not required to do or think about anything else. This can involve doing absolutely nothing, listening to music, reading a book or so on.

Exercise is one way of relaxing, as long as you don't find exercise stressful in itself. It, of course, has the added effect of keeping you fit as well. Even a brisk mile or so walk a day may make a noticeable difference.

Floatation Tanks

Using a floatation tank involves lying naked or in a swimming costume in a tank of salt water, with both the air and water at body temperature. The tank is covered so that you are lying in pitch black. All external stimuli are therefore stopped, and this enables your brain to relax. The whole procedure lasts about one hour and is said to have some amazing relaxing effects.

Hypnotherapy

Hypnotherapy is much more than relaxation. It aims to get right to the bottom of your problems and clear them, rather than being, perhaps, a more superficial treatment. More can be seen about this in the psychology chapter.

Massage

Massage can be very helpful, especially if done using aromatherapy oils. It is certainly worth trying, many people find that they can give a massage without needing any further instructions, others find that a bit of direction is needed.

Meditation

The aim of meditation is to reach a level of rest and relaxation that is better than that attained through sleep. It is essential to meditate regularly, ideally twice a day for about twenty minutes each time. This will lead to an increasingly relaxing effect. In addition, it will be easier to go to sleep, and you should feel that you need less sleep. Concentration also improves and you generally feel better. To begin with, concentrating on the meditation itself will be difficult, but it will come with practice.

There are a variety of ways to meditate and you should really find the method that best suits you. You must sit or lie in a comfortable position, with no distractions. You should take deep, gentle breaths into the abdomen.

One method is to concentrate on counting your breaths, going from one to ten and then starting from one again. Another method is to visualise your breath coming into your body and then out again.

A further method is to visualise a simple object, or think of a simple word and concentrate on this or to listen to a regular sound, such as the ticking of a clock.

A version of this method is to concentrate on the number one until you get distracted, then to go on to number two, then three and so on.

This method has the additional advantage of being able to track your progress, so will give you confidence to continue, if you feel that after a week or so of meditating you have not improved. You will find that the number of distractions that occur in your meditation period will slowly reduce.

There are various adjustments on these themes, and a little experimentation will be necessary to find what suits you best.

Relaxation Training

Relaxation training is a method of progressive relaxation that involves tensing and relaxing muscles.

Self-hypnosis

Self-hypnosis is becoming increasingly popular. It involves visualising a relaxing scene such as being in the country or by the seaside and concentrating on this. Nowadays, there are many cassettes and videos that are available which can help you do this. Some of these have subliminal messages that are recorded, but you cannot actually hear them. They do, however, have a further relaxing effect.

Stress Management

Stress management is a method of handling stress that involves a variety of the techniques discussed in this book. This tends to be done as a group therapy rather than an individual therapy.

Tai Chi Chuan

Tai chi is a martial art that concentrates more on relaxation, concentration and balance than on self defence. It is a form of healing, a form of self defence and a spiritual discipline.

Yoga

Yoga is much more than just a relaxation exercise. It involves attaining a certain connection between the mind and body that gives you more control over yourself. There are a variety of mind and body exercises involved in order to do this. The Yoga for Health Foundation say that they have had a few people with epilepsy to stay and all have shown some level of improvement.

Yoga can be very complex to learn completely and will take a number of years. However, it is also fairly easy to begin and to notice some improvement from. If you want to learn it thoroughly it is probably necessary to go on a short course. However, a lot can be learnt from a book and this will certainly enable you to get a feel for it and decide if you like it.

Case Study

Sarah was injured at school during a hockey match and this brought on her epilepsy. What with the epilepsy itself and the drugs as well, she was confined to a wheelchair and having fits very regularly. However, after an intensive yoga course she managed to get a control over the epilepsy and is now completely recovered.

Chapter 5 – Chiropractice, Osteopathy and Cranial Massage

Introduction

Chiropractice and osteopathy involve the manipulation of the vertebrae of the spine to correct any imbalances. If the vertebrae are incorrectly positioned, the nerves that run through them may be damaged or pushed out of shape, which could lead to them behaving incorrectly. Therefore the aim is to ensure that there is no interference in the body's nerve supply.

There are various forms of cranial massage that tend to come under slightly different names. The aims of the different kinds of massage are much the same: to release pressure and ensure that the various parts of the skull and brain are correctly positioned.

I have heard of a few people who have been helped by chiropractice and osteopathy. In some cases, just one treatment cured them.

Causes

There are many causes of different problems that can be helped by chiropractice or osteopathy. The causes include both giving birth and being born, falls and accidents, emotional stress, poor posture, an unsuitable mattress and so on. If it is obvious that your problem has started because one or more of these circumstances, it is certainly worth considering a chiropractor. It is also possible for vertebrae to move after a very slight accident of which you might not have taken any notice or even remember.

Symptoms

In cases of epilepsy, misalignments will occur at the very top of the spine. Other symptoms that may occur in this case are headaches, nervousness, insomnia, head colds, high blood pressure, migraines, mental conditions, nervous breakdowns, amnesia, sleeping sickness, chronic tiredness, dizziness or vertigo, St Vitus dance, sinus troubles, allergies, crossed eyes, deafness, erysipelas, eye troubles, earache, fainting spells, some blindness. Therefore if you feel that you suffer from any of these, it may well be worth seeing a chiropractor, and you may find that the root of your problem is purely a slightly misaligned vertebrae.

Chiropractice versus Osteopathy

Although there are some differences between chiropractice and osteopathy, the two seem to be slowly merging. The main difference is that a chiropractor tends to use short, sharp thrusts to realign the displaced vertebrae, whereas an osteopath may use more gentle rotation and stretching of limbs.

Cranial Massage

Cranial massage involves adjusting the different bones in the skull into their correct positions. When a child is born the bones in the head are unattached, this makes birth easier because they can adjust and move in order to fit the birth canal. In time, these bones slowly join together although they are never firmly fixed.

In most cases these bones then move back into their correct place as the child grows. Unfortunately this does not always happen. Failure to do this can lead to brain damage, cerebral palsy, autism, dyslexia, epilepsy, behavioural and personality disorders and many other related problems. In severe cases the problem may be obvious from birth, especially if the skull is visibly deformed, but in many other cases it may take years before the problem comes to light.

Cranial massage therapy is like a very gentle massage and so can be used on babies, old people and those who are very delicate. It is most effective on babies since that is when the skull is most pliable. In fact, it is possibly something that should be considered with every child who suffers from fits from birth or very soon afterwards.

Although the bones are much more adaptable in children and young adults, it can help in older people as well, although perhaps not to the same degree. It is important to get this sort of problem treated as soon as possible.

Treating Yourself

It is not possible to treat yourself, or get a friend to treat you, with any of the above therapies, since quite a lot of training is required before you are suitably experienced.

Case Studies

Debbie started having fits when she was six months old. The fits were very frequent, at times every few minutes. She was taken into hospital and given the usual treatments, but nothing seemed to help. A cranial osteopath visited her in hospital, and after one treatment her condition had improved amazingly and she was allowed to return home. At the time of writing she was still undergoing treatment.

Apparently she had been a very difficult birth and her head had been forced back a long way. This had caused the bones of the scalp and neck to move out of place and had therefore triggered off the attacks.

Chapter 6 – Low Blood Sugar

Introduction

Low blood sugar is also known as hypoglycaemia. Some people consider that over half the population have this problem. The symptoms are considerably varied and include both physical and psychological types. If your epilepsy is triggered by this, then the easiest way of telling is that your fits will generally happen when you have an empty stomach. Therefore they are most likely to be in the morning before having breakfast. They are also likely to be more frequent when under stress. If you have a history of diabetes in the family, or are a sugar addict, then it is more probable that you have a blood sugar problem, and it is also more important that you do something about it.

There has been an amazing increase in the occurrence of hypoglycaemia in the last century, which is due to the increase in processed food, especially sugar. The traditional test for hypo-glycaemia is to go without food and only drink water for twelve hours. You then take some glucose and your blood is tested at regular intervals for the level of glucose in the blood. However, alternative medicine believes that the level at which there is a problem is much lower than that at which conventional medicine believes there is a problem. Also, the level at which there can be a problem may depend on the individual and may not be noticeable in a test. This means that if you are given the test by a conventional practitioner he may say that you have not got a problem, when in fact you have. On the other hand, if this is the case then, you will only have a mild version of the problem.

How to Tell if you Suffer from Low Blood Sugar

The most obvious symptom is that you feel very much worse on an empty stomach. Other likely symptoms are a severe lack of energy, a

47

craving for sweets and sugar, a desire to eat when perhaps you are not hungry and a range of psychological problems that perhaps seem to come and go. For instance, sometimes you may be depressed or angry for no obvious reason at all, and then it may go and you feel quite happy. Mood swings are very common. Bad cases can lead to suicidal tendencies, extreme violence and other similar problems. You may feel that you think you have severe psychological problems, when it is purely an imbalance in the body. It also seems that many people who suffer from low blood sugar also suffer from allergies.

If you find that your condition improves when you are pregnant, then this is another symptom that the problem may be due to low blood sugar. However, you may also experience the matter getting worse when you are pregnant. The pancreas is situated just below the left rib, and you may find that this is rather tender if you have a blood sugar problem.

Reason

The pancreas produces insulin to keep the level of blood sugar in the body stable. However, the use of processed sugar is a relatively recent development and the pancreas was not designed to cope with this. Eating sugar means that there is a sudden increase in blood sugar, as opposed to the gradual one from any other type of carbohydrate, and the pancreas has to react fast in order to handle this. In time the pancreas tends to get worn out because it has been over used, it doesn't work as efficiently as it used to and can, in the long term, lead to diabetes. Treatment involves the reduction of the changes in the blood sugar level and assistance to the pancreas to help it do its job properly. This can counteract the problem completely, although it does not always happen immediately. I have also heard of people successfully using the treatment below to gain a cure for diabetes.

In the past, the treatment given was to have sugar whenever you felt tired or weak, but in time it was realised that this didn't get to the root of the problem and could actually make things worse.

Treatment

Treatment of low blood sugar can be handled fairly well without going to a practitioner. There are many books available on the topic, and it is worth reading some of them. Most libraries will have at least one book on the topic. The only problem with reading many books is that they all tend to recommend slightly different things and the more you read, the more you may get confused.

Basically the treatment can be split into two types: one for those who suffer severely and one for those who suffer mildly. In all cases you may find that, when you start the treatment, for a couple of weeks you feel very tired. This is a good thing is as much as it proves that low blood sugar levels is a problem with you and that some treatment is necessary. This tiredness occurs because your pancreas needs to adjust to the different level of sugar intake.

The most severe treatment involves the complete elimination of sugar from the diet. Initially the diet will exclude dried fruit, honey, bananas and large quantities of other fruit. Bread, pasta and other flour based products should only be made from wholemeal flour. Brown bread and other similar products do not count – if it does not say wholemeal then it is not. Wholemeal flour is the only flour that is not allowed to have chemicals added to it, and is better for you because it is ground from the full grain. Similarly, wholegrain rice should be used, rather than white or processed rice. If you don't think that your problem is so severe, then try cutting down on sugar. Complete elimination of sugar is not essential. Do try hard to stick to wholemeal flour. Coffee, tobacco and alcohol should be avoided, and bananas should only be eaten in moderation.

It is also important to try to eat regularly. Every three hours is ideal, although this may only be a snack. However with a bit of practice you should be able to tell when you need food. Some days will be worse than others. Slowly you will be able to adjust your diet to the way you feel each day.

There are many supplements recommended for the treatment of blood sugar problems. Often it is not practical to take them all but there are a few that are essential. Further information can be found in the chapter on vitamins and minerals.

B COMPLEX

This has two functions. Firstly B vitamins help considerably under stress conditions. Secondly, they help the stability of the adrenal glands, pancreas and liver. A high supplement of this can be very helpful. It is very difficult to overdose on B vitamins but if your urine turns yellow this shows that your body is rejecting the excess and therefore does not need any more. It is not a problem, but just signifies that there is no point in having any more.

BREWER'S YEAST

Some people reckon that a regular dose of brewer's yeast can get rid of low blood sugar problems in many people, with no other supplements needed. This is certainly worth a try since brewer's yeast is not very expensive and has a yeasty flavour that very few people dislike. It is high in the B vitamins and in chromium.

VITAMIN C

This is used up at a considerable level when under stress and also when the adrenal glands are overworked. This means that under these circumstances, there is a very high possibility of going down with colds and infections, so a supplement is useful. It also helps stabilise insulin production. Very large quantities of vitamin C can lead to diarrhoea, although they have no lasting side effects.

CALCIUM

This helps the processing of the B vitamins. Calcium should also be taken if a supplement of magnesium is taken.

CHROMIUM

This is regularly used in the treatment of low blood sugar. The recommended form is that labelled GTF or glucose tolerance factor, but all chromium will be very helpful. It also helps with high cholesterol levels.

VITAMIN E

It has also been shown to help the uptake of glucose.

LECITHIN

This is a good source of choline, which is a member of the B complex, and also of phosphorus.

MAGNESIUM

This helps the liver to do its job and is known to help low blood sugar.

POTASSIUM

When under stress, large amounts of potassium can be lost. Additional potassium can help regulate the blood sugar.

RAW ADRENAL

The adrenal glands produce an anti-stress hormone. Since stress can upset the blood sugar level, adrenal supplements can help to stabilise this.

RAW PANCREAS

This supplement will increase the volume of the enzymes produced by the pancreas to stabilise the blood sugar.

SPIRULINA

This is a type of seaweed which is very high in nutrients.

ZINC

This can delay the absorption of glucose and helps to regulate insulin release. Supplementation should be in range 25-50mg.

If you follow the above diet for about four to six weeks and find that there is no change, then check that you are following the rules correctly. Many things such as vitamin and mineral supplements can have sugar added and not say so. Therefore make sure that you take supplements which have no sugar added to them. Some foods that you didn't check could have added sugar – it is amazing what sugar is added to. If you still show no improvement then it is probably worth trying a different treatment. Although improvement will occur within a month or so, further improvements may occur at a much later time as well.

Chapter 7 – Detoxification

Introduction

Detoxification is necessary when the body has an excessive build up of toxins, and this can show itself in many forms, including epilepsy. These toxins can be of various types and are generally chemical based, especially in epilepsy. Pesticides and other chemicals used in the production of foods can cause a build up of toxins in the system, and some people are particularly sensitive to this. For this reason it is a good idea to avoid as many chemicals in food and the environment as possible.

Heavy Metal Toxins

Fits can also be affected by excess aluminium, copper, chemicals and pesticides. The simplest way to reduce these is to get a water filter. The sort of filter that is relatively cheap and can be got from most health food shops will remove many of the metals and some of the other chemicals, as well as making the water taste better. If the water is a problem with you, you may find that the quantity of fits is affected by where you are and therefore what water you are drinking.

It is not just foods that can trigger fits, chemicals in the air can have an effect as well. For instance, some paints or air fresheners can have effects. So can medicines. If your fits have occurred when on a specific type of drug, is it likely that you are allergic to this?

If you live in an area where the air is not very clear, you may find that this has some effect. This is particularly likely if you have breathing problems. If the air does affect you, probably you will find that you are much worse in humid weather and much better if you go into the country. However, one or two days in the country may just cause you to cough, have a mild dose of diarrhoea or something like that, since the body has to clear the toxins from the system before it can start feeling better.

Symptoms of Toxification

Epilepsy, can be caused by an excess of aluminium, lead or mercury in the system, along with overdoses of many other chemicals.

Patients suffering from lead poisoning will tend to be those who have a lot of contact with car fumes, those who drive a lot on main roads, or those who live in inner cities. If you suffer from lead toxification you probably will find that the condition gets worse when the atmosphere is very humid. Lead toxification is more common in children, and so it is important to keep them away from lead toys and other lead products. Convulsions may be a sign that there is a problem before it gets to any sort of danger level, since it is one of the first symptoms. A mild anaemia is also a fairly early symptom as is mental disturbance. The condition may be an acute case of a sudden intake of lead for one reason or another. In this case it will go away on its own in a fairly short period of time, although following some of the recommendations in this chapter will definitely speed this improvement. If you follow these procedures, you are helping nature do its job and so there should be no after effects at all, although it is possible that there is a temporary worsening of the condition.

The most likely sufferers of mercury poisoning are those who have many fillings in their teeth, or whose condition gets noticeably worse, after they have had fillings. As above, mercury poisoning can occur as a short acute condition, due to a temporary excess intake or can occur as a chronic condition due to a slow build up over a period of time. As with lead poisoning, convulsions are one of the earlier symptoms. By the time more symptoms appear it should be obvious to any doctor that mercury poisoning has occurred.

Below is a list of many of the symptoms which can occur when the body has too high an intake of aluminium, lead or mercury.

	Symptoms	Causes	
Aluminium	Alzheimer's disease	Baking powder	
	Behavioural disfunction	Beer cans	
	Brain degeneration	Construction materials	
	Colic	Cookware	
	Digestive disorders	Deodorants	
	Gastritis	Emulsifier in cheese	
	Headache	Salt	
	Kidney disorders		
	Motor dysfunction		
	Seizures		
	Skin rash		
Lead	Anaemia	Car exhaust	Most common in small children, who are nearer the ground and hence most susceptible to car fumes.
	Appetite loss	Cigarettes	Absorption of lead is reduced when there is an adequate intake of zinc and calcium.
	Arthritis	Cooking utensils	
	Ataxia	Hair colourings	
	Birth defects	Lead paint	
	Cataracts	Lead pipes in soft water areas	
	Concentration	Newspaper ink	
	Confusion	Organ meats	
	Constipation	Pesticides	
	Depression	Shellfish	
	Digestion problems	Smelters	
	Emotional instability		
	Fatigue		
	Gout		
	Headaches		
	Hyperactivity		
	Hypertension		
	Impotence		
	Insomnia		
	Irritability		
	Kidney damage		
	Learning difficulties		
	Liver cirrhosis		
	Metallic taste		
	Motor neuron degeneration		
	Muscle aches & weakness		

	Nausea		
	Pituitary damage		
	Restlessness		
	Schizophrenic behaviour		
	Seizures		
	Thyroid dysfunction		
	Tremors		
	Vertigo		
	Vomiting		
Mercury	Abdominal pain	Cosmetics	If you have many dental fillings it may be worth getting checked out, the cheapest way is with a hair analysis test.
	Birth defects	Dental fillings	
	Chromosome damage	Drugs	
	Fatigue	Fabric softeners	
	Gingivitis	Fertilisers	
	Headaches	Fungicides	Can contribute to all diseases.
	Hearing loss	Pesticides	
	Insanity	Pollution	
	Kidney damage	Water based paints	
	Mental retardation		
	Nausea		
	Nervousness		
	Seizures		
	Skin eruptions		
	Sore gums		
	Tooth loss		
	Tremors		
	Vertigo		
	Vision loss		
	Vomiting		

Detoxification

The basis of detoxification is to reduce the body's intake of toxins as much as possible, and at the same time to increase the body's elimination processes as much as possible. This method can be followed intensely over a short period of time, or more gently over a

56

longer period. Since the intensive method can sometimes have a violent effect, which may cause a short term increase in fits, I would recommend the longer but slower method.

There are a variety of detoxification diets which are written about in books and magazines. To a certain extent, the best is the one which you feel is most suitable for you, but they do all tend to be very similar.

Tests back at the beginning of the century showed that many epileptics stopped having fits when they were fasting, although this is obviously no long term solution to the problem; it is the basis that many of the detoxification diets work on, and the foods which are eliminated in the diets listed below are those which tend to lead to fits, and other problems, when eaten.

Vitamins and Other Nutrients for Detoxification

The nutrients listed below are those that are most recommended for detoxification, for further information on them see the vitamin and mineral section.

VITAMIN C

This is known to be a detoxifier and can be given in large quantities of up to 6g a day, spread out over the day. If diarrhoea should result then decrease the dosage.

CALCIUM

Calcium decreases the absorption of heavy metals. However, extra milk should not be taken since this can increase lead levels.

GARLIC

Garlic is often recommended for increasing the workings of the body, and it assists elimination processes.

MAGNESIUM

Magnesium helps to repair body cells, so it will help reduce any damage which has occurred from the build up of toxins

MANGANESE

Manganese is very good for the nervous system and for elimination. It should be taken with zinc supplements of over 50mg.

SELENIUM

Selenium protects against toxic substances and also help liver function and therefore elimination through the liver.

ZINC

Zinc has a variety of functions, including the elimination of toxins.

Gerson Therapy

One common, and perhaps the most severe detoxification process is the Gerson Therapy. It was designed by Max Gerson during the Second World War. Its main use was as a treatment of cancer but it has been successful in treating many other conditions, including epilepsy.

The basis of the therapy is to remove all the toxins from the body. This is done by taking a diet very high in vegetables and fruit juices and by the regular use of enemas. This is a very severe diet and generally is only necessary with acute conditions where it is obviously essential to rid the body of toxins as fast as possible. Cancer is a typical example of this; it generally cannot be left for very long since the condition will get worse, maybe at a very fast rate. However, in the case of epilepsy it is somewhat different. Epilepsy seldom gets noticeably worse to a degree when life is endangered, although this is not unknown. This therapy also requires a lot of time, to the degree of being a full time job. To most people, this uses up more time than is available and therefore is completely impractical. One further problem is that, when a severe improvement to the diet occurs suddenly it can make the condition worse for a short length of time, while many of the toxins are eliminated from the body. Therefore, for the average epileptic who is interested in experimenting with this diet, the best procedure is probably to do the changes slowly and to do only those parts that you feel comfortable with and that you can manage to keep up over a longish period of time, ideally a few months.

The Full Diet

It is important when following the diet to concentrate on the freshness of all the food and also do your best to ensure that it is salt and fat free.

Breakfast consists of organic oats mixed 1:3 with water and with added fruit. The added fruit can be any fruit other than berries and pineapples; dried fruits should not be sulphur treated. Some sweetener is allowed in the porridge and this must be in the form of the darkest Barbados sugar, light honey, black strap molasses or pure maple syrup containing no formaldehyde.

Lunch and dinner consist of a salad that can use a wide variety of vegetables and a choice of dressings, followed by a cup of special vegetable soup.

A large quantity of juices are taken with the diet: orange juice, carrot and apple juice made from equal quantities of carrots and apples, green juice made from all kinds of lettuce – endive, red cabbage and green pepper – and liver juice made from fresh calves liver. These juices must be prepared freshly.

With the exception of liver juice, goat yoghurt is the only animal product that is allowed in the diet. This is not normally taken until a few months into the diet.

A variety of medications are taken. The aim of these is to encourage the body to remove the toxins. These medications include

59

potassium, iodine, pancreatic enzymes and pepsin.

Enemas are also given in order to help remove all the toxins from the body, which have been brought to the surface by the diet.

Macrobiotic Diet

The macrobiotic diet is becoming increasingly more popular. Generally it is not used so much as a treatment, but more as a long term change in diet in order to improve health. It involves the elimination of all processed foods, sugar, caffeine, alcohol, dairy products and meat, though fish is allowed if wanted. Although this may sound practically impossible, it is not that difficult, once you have got a good recipe book.

As above, it is perhaps not a good idea to suddenly have a complete change of diet. You may find it much easier to introduce it over a period of time. Of course, it is also not essential to stick to it completely, but you will undoubtedly feel an improvement in your general health, if not your fits and you may find that in time you do not want to eat anything else.

Self Treatment

If you want to follow either diet to the full, it is almost essential to get some advice from a qualified nutritional therapy practitioner. This is partly because they will be able to give you various advice that you would not be able to get from books alone, and they will be able to relate the treatment to your specific condition. Also, you are likely to experience healing crises, which are times when you will feel particularly ill, as the body tries to eliminate the toxins from the body. This is rather like developing a cough when you give up smoking and the body is trying to remove all the rubbish from your lungs.

Although these diets are very severe and very strict for those people with severe conditions, in mild cases it is a good idea to experiment with one of them and take it gently and only as far as you feel that you can manage it. For instance, you could start by cutting out coffee and then when you are happy with this you could cut out red meat and so on. Another possibility is, for example, to go on a diet of only raw fruit and vegetables for three days, or even to fast, although the latter is only recommended if you are generally in good health.

PART 2

Methods of Treatment

Chapter 8 – Aromatherapy

Introduction

Aromatherapy is the use of essential oils to improve your health and general wellbeing. These can be applied in various ways, the most common of them with massage. Many people use the aromatherapy oils at home either by evaporating them in burners or by adding them to the bath. Some of the oils can be taken internally in very small doses, but this should only be done when recommended by a qualified practitioner. Aromatherapy can be used for general first aid as well.

Aromatherapy in Relation to Epilepsy

The majority of aromatherapy oils can be divided into two groups: those that stimulate and those that relax. Since epilepsy tends to be stress related, those oils that are used to relax people are those that are used to treat epilepsy. Relief from the fits may not be achieved from the use of aromatherapy alone, even though it often is. However, acceptance of the difficulties involved is often managed and people who use aromatherapy tend to find themselves more relaxed and able to handle what life throws at them.

There are many oils that can be used to help epilepsy, and to a certain extent it will depend on the individual as to which are the most effective. Since everybody has different health problems the oils should be selected that will best cover all your health problems. For instance, chamomile may be used if you also suffer from anaemia, whereas rosemary will be used if you also suffer from rheumatism. A fairly reliable way of selecting oils is by selecting the aromas that appeal to you. They will almost certainly work for you too. However, it is also important to be aware that some oils can cause convulsions and that many should not be used on pregnant or lactating women.

Aromatherapy on the Cheap

It is definitely a good idea to see a qualified practitioner of aromatherapy (see addresses in Appendix 1) at least for a few times, so that they can give you directions about what you can do for yourself. However, if you would like to play around a little at home, a good starter is a bottle of lavender oil. This is one of the cheapest available – some of the oils can be very expensive because they are difficult to produce. Put about five drops of lavender oil in a bath that is fairly full, but not too hot, and lay in it for about half an hour and you should feel noticeably more relaxed. Clary sage is another oil that is very helpful: it does wonders for depression. If you want to try the use of massage you can add a few drops of the essential oil to a quantity of cooking oil and rub it into your skin. There are many oils that are better than ordinary cooking oil – such as almond oil and olive oil – but this will at least give you some idea of what aromatherapy is all about, without having to pay out extra money. There are many books available on aromatherapy both in bookshops and libraries and it may be well worth your while reading one of these.

Oils to Help Epilepsy

Various experiments have been done using aromatherapy on epileptics. Melissa and chamomile have been found to lead to a substantial decrease in the number of fits.

Essential Oil	Other Conditions Helped	Warnings
Angelica	Skin and digestive	Avoid if pregnant or diabetic
Aniseed	Infections	Avoid if suffering from skin conditions
Lemon Balm	Skin	
French Basil	Nervous system	Avoid during pregnancy
West Indian Bay	Skin, hair and muscular	Use in moderation
Bergamot	Skin and nervous system	
Cardamom	Digestive	

Cedarwood	Skin and respiratory system	Use in moderation, avoid during pregnancy
Chamomile	Skin	
Cinammon	Digestive and nervous system	
Coriander	Accumulation of fluids and toxins	Use in moderation
Cumin	Digestive and nervous system	Avoid during pregnancy
Cypress	Skin and muscles	
Dill	Digestive system, lack of periods	
Eucalyptus	Skin, muscular and respiratory	
Ginger	Circulation and digestive	
Hops	Nervous system, female problems	Avoid during depression
Jasmine	Depression and stress related	
Juniper	Muscular and circulation	Use in moderation
Lavender	Skin and nervous system	
Lemon	Skin and circulation	Use in moderation
Lovage	Circulation and joints	Avoid during pregnancy
Mandarin	Nervous system	
Marjoram	Nervous system and muscular	Avoid during pregnancy
Mint	Respiratory system	
Niaouli	Respiratory system and skin	
Orange Blossom	Skin and nervous system	
Black Pepper	Muscles and circulation	Use in moderation
Rose	Skin and female problems	
Rosewood	Skin	
Clary Sage	Skin and nervous system	Avoid during pregnancy and when drinking alcohol
Sandalwood	Skin and respiratory system	
Savory		Don't use on skin
Tarragon	Digestive system, female problems	Avoid during pregnancy
Thyme	Skin and respiratory system	Avoid during pregnancy
Valerian	Nervous system	Use in moderation
Lemon Verbena	Digestive and nervous systems	
Ylang ylang	Skin and nervous system	Use in moderation

Oils to be Avoided

The main oils that should be avoided by epileptics are fennel, hyssop, rosemary and sage. Rosemary is on this list despite the fact that it has been shown to help with epilepsy. However, it should only be used by a qualified aromatherapist as some people can be very susceptible.

Treating Yourself

Above, is a list of oils which are known to help epilepsy. In order to find the oils most suited to your requirements, select those which list other problems which you may have in the Other Conditions Helped column. Most people will have some problems in this column, however slight. Remember to take notice of the information in the warning column. When you have done this, ignore the ones which you know that you do not like the smell of. This will give you a fairly short list of oils. The price of the different oils can vary considerably, so obviously this can play a part in the selection of oils. Some oils are much more easily obtainable than others. You should end up with about three or four oils, which can be used in the methods mentioned above.

Professional Treatment

A professional aromatherapist will be able to make a much better decision as to which oils are suitable for your particular problems. All your health problems, large or small, will be taken into consideration and the oils from the above list, and various others, which best suit your problems will be selected. These will normally be applied in the form of a massage, on a weekly basis. The frequency of the treatments can be reduced as your condition improves. The practitioner will obviously be able to give you any necessary advice and answer any questions that you may have. A great deal of research is being done into aromatherapy as a treatment for epilepsy by Tim Betts at the University of Birmingham.

Case Studies

One recent study was carried out by Teena Clouston and was included in the International Journal of Aromatherapy for Autumn 1991. She treated people with complex partial seizures by giving them a twenty minute back massage. She found melissa especially useful for one young woman who was suffering from a high incidence of pre-menstrual seizures. Chamomile was used for one middle aged woman and it led to a 90% reduction in seizures.

Chapter 9 – Homoeopathy

Introduction

Homoeopathy is one of the more recognised forms of alternative treatments. Homoeopathic treatment is preferred by many because it is the most similar to conventional medicine, in that it consists of taking certain tablets at certain times. However, the concepts behind homoeopathy are completely different to those behind conventional medicine.

Homoeopathy, like many forms of complementary medicine, believes that the symptoms are the body's reaction against the illness, rather than being caused by the illness, as conventional medicine does. This requires a somewhat different approach to that of conventional medicine. Homoeopathic treatment aims to help encourage the body to stabilise this imbalance and therefore get rid of the illness.

The remedies used in homoeopathy are minute traces of substances which cause symptoms similar to what is at the root of the problem. This has the effect of strengthening the body against the problem.

When prescribing, the homoeopath will take into consideration many things as well as the main problem, for instance, whether you are an excitable person, whether you get indigestion and so on. The conditions under which you have fits and the nature of them will be particularly important. This enables the homoeopath to produce a treatment that is tailormade to the individual and which is best able to correct any imbalance.

Below is a list of the different homoeopathic treatments used to treat epilepsy.

Remedy		Treatment
Arg Nit Argentum Nitricum Silver Nitrate	Character	Anxious Fearful of being alone Fearful of public speaking Hurried Impulsive Weak memory
	Symptoms	Exhaustion with trembling Cravings for sugar Face sallow Needle like pains Sour taste in mouth Red tipped tongue Diarrhoea Eye inflammation Flatulence Headache Hoarseness Indigestion Sore throat
	Better for	Fresh air Company Bathing in cold water
	Worse for	Heat After eating sweets and sugar Cold food Cold air Thinking intently
Caulophyllum Papoose Root Squaw root Blueberry root	Symptoms	Joint pain Labour pain
	Better for	Heat Closed spaces
	Worse for	Cold Open air Coffee
Causticum Potassium Hydrate	Character	Restless Absent minded

Tinctura acris sine kali		Anxious
		Depressed
		Irritable
		Sympathetic
		Fearful
	Symptoms	Blister on tip of tongue
		Red stripe down middle with white edges of tongue
		Clumsy
		Heavy eyelids
		Likes smoked foods
		Poor concentration
		Tearful
		Constipation
		Cough
		Cramp
		Hoarseness
		Indigestion
		Joint pain
		Sore throat
		Respiratory problems
		Urinary Problems
	Better for	Cold drinks
		Heat
		Warmth of bed
		Damp wet weather
	Worse for	Changes in weather
		Coffee
		Cold
		Draughts
		During evening
		Fresh air
		Walking
		Getting wet
Cicuta	Symptoms	Concussion
		Spasms
	Better for	Warmth
	Worse for	Touch
		Draughts
		Tobacco smoke

Cocculus	Symptoms	Sensation of emptiness or hollowness
		Intense dislike of contradiction
		Time passes quickly
		Seasickness
		Giddiness with nausea
		Aversion to food even when looking at it
		Desire for cold drinks
	Better for	Being in a warm room
		Lying quiet
	Worse for	Eating
		Drinking
		Smoking
		Talking
		Motion of ship
Crotalus	Character	Suspicious
		Forgetful
	Better for	Inside
		Coolness
	Worse for	Open air
		Damp
		Heat
		Sleep
		Hot drinks
Cuprum	Character	Anxious
	Symptoms	Shortness of breath
		Hysteria
		Cramps
		Asthma
	Better for	Perspiration
		Cold water
	Worse for	Night
		Before menstruation
		Being sick
Glonomium	Character	Confused
	Symptoms	Dizziness
		Headaches

	Better for	Cold air
		Cold applications
		Bending head back
		Lying with head higher than hips
	Worse for	Heat
		Exertion
		Noise
		Sunlight
		Bright light
		Wine
		Stimulants
		Tight clothes
Ignatia	Character	Children-Bright
		-Precocious
		-Highly Strung
		Adults-Alert
		-Nervous
		-Rather pale
	Symptoms	Headaches
		Sensitivity to pain
		Sore throat
	Better for	Eating
		Urinating
		From pressure
		Walking
		External heat
	Worse for	Fear
		Anxiety
		Fresh air
		Cold
		Coffee
		Brandy
Nux vomica	Character	Self reliance
		Efficiency
		A liking for hard work
	Symptoms	Hangovers
		Headaches
		Aching muscles
	Better for	Warmth

		Sleep
		Pressure
	Worse for	Cold
		Wind
		Dryness
		Noise
		Spices
		Stimulants
		Eating
		Getting angry
Plumbum	Character	Melancholy
		Indifference
		Depression
	Symptoms	Lead posioning
	Better for	Rubbing
		Hard pressure
		Physical exertion
	Worse for	At night
		Motion
Pulsatilla Wind Flower	Character	Timid and fearful
		Mild and gentle
		Silent and melancholic
		Easily moved to laughter and tears
	Symptoms	Secretion from all mucous membranes are thick, blank and yellowish green
		Nothing tastes good
		Absense of thirst
		Repugnance to food
		Chilly yet averse to heat
		Symptoms ever changing
		Gastric complaints from rich food
		Periods delayed and irregular
	Better for	Cold
		Fresh open air
		Gentle motion
		Erect posture

		A good cry
		Rubbing
		Lying with head high
	Worse for	Warmth
		Warm closed room
		Getting wet feet
		In evening
		Rest
		Motion
		Eating rich foods
		Puberty
		Pregnancy

There are many homoeopathic cures now available from health food shops and chemists. Unfortunately, although these are very useful for simple conditions it may be difficult to treat something like epilepsy yourself. However, if you are interested in trying this it may be worth reading a book on the topic. Homoeopathy possibly has more books in the local libraries than any other branch of alternative medicine, so it should be fairly easy to find something that is suitable.

The above chart should enable you to get a better idea of which remedy is most suitable. Look down the lists of characters and symptoms and find one that best suits your condition. All of the above homoeopathic remedies can be used to help epilepsy, but to find the correct one for the individual treatment, it is necessary to match up other character details and symptoms. It is then necessary to find the suitable remedy. Some are available in most health food shops, others are not so easily accessible; in this case it may be worth contacting some of the addresses in Appendix 1. It is also possible to get prescriptions for homoeopathic remedies from some doctors. It is very important to follow the instructions on the jar. Don't take more or less than the quantity recommended and don't mix remedies. If you find that it does not have any effect, maybe try a different remedy. You should find that the treatment will not only help the epilepsy, but also will help various other minor ailments.

It is possible that the condition will get slightly worse when you start taking homoeopathic treatments. This shows that they are working. If it does happen then stop taking the pills until this aggravation has passed and then retake them.

Case Studies

Sally was 18 when she started being given homoeopathic treatment. She had had severe measles at the age of 13. When she started menstruating, she had a fit with almost every period, and the fit was always preceded by a very bad headache. She was given glonoine with the onset of the headache and the fits stopped.

Alan was 36, he had severe fits, usually in the afternoon. He was give zinc phosphate and had an almost complete cure.

Chapter 10 – Herbal Treatment

Introduction

Herbs have been used for the treatment of ailments for many thousands of years. They are included in many of the old wives treatments, and many conventional treatments are based on the old herbal treatments. They certainly have many uses and can be very helpful. Generally, they are taken in one of two forms, either as tea or as capsules. There are a great many herbs that are helpful in stress-related conditions.

The herbs used are a range of plants, not necessarily what you would consider herbs in the cooking sense. As in other forms of treatment you can treat yourself or go to a practitioner. If you intend to treat yourself it is usually a good idea to take a book out of the library on the topic. It also may be worth seeing a local practitioner for a bit of advice on a one off basis before you start or when you have been experimenting for a little while.

Treating Yourself

There are many herbs that are available from the shops, some addresses are in the Appendix. In order to make them into teas, the general procedure is to put one to two teaspoons of the herb in a cupful of boiling water and leave it to infuse for about ten minutes. Below is a list of herbs that can be used. Go through and decide which ones you think are most suitable for your situation. A combination of herbs can be used, and is often better.

Herb	Further Details
Black cohosh	Stimulates and normalises menstrual flow
	Gradually restores the proper function of the body
	Sedative and anti-spasmodic
Catnip Nepeta cataria	Helps digestion and reduces gas
	Aids the skin in elimination of toxins
	Contracts tissues and hence reduces secretions and discharges
	Sedative and anti-spasmodic
Cayenne	Helps digestion and reduces gas
	Increase blood circulation in skin and can relieve internal pains
	Stimulates the secretion of saliva
	Stimulant, tonic and antiseptic
Chamomile Anthemis Nobilis	Helps heal wounds and cuts
	Reduces pain
	Helps digestion and reduces gas
	Anti-spasmodic, anti-septic, anti-inflammatory
Gotu kola Hydrocotle Indian Pennywort	Restorative and relaxant for nervous system
	Diuretic
	Locally healing and cleansing
Hyssop Hyssopus officinalis	For use with petit mal
	Helps digestion and reduces gas
	Encourages the elimination of toxins through the skin
	Anti-spasmodic, expectorant and sedative
Lady's Slipper	Strengthens the nervous system
	Sedative, hypnotic, anti-spasmodic and tonic
Lobelia Lobelia inflata	Take at first sign of fit
	Causes vomiting
	Respiratory stimulant, anti-asthmatic, anti-spasmodic and expectorant
Loranthus	This is based on mistletoe grown on the wild oak
	Anti-spasmodic
Mistletoe	Strengthens nervous system
	Cardiac depressant and possibly anti-tumour
Mugwort	For menstrual cycle related epilepsy
	Stimulates and normalises menstrual flow
	Strengthens nervous system
	Bitter tonic and stimulant

Passion Flower Passiflora incarnata	Pain killer, sedative, hypnotic and anti-spasmodic
Peony root Paeonia officinalis	Anti-spasmodic, diuretic, sedative Helps kidney and bladder problems Be careful – the flowers are fatal
Skullcap Scutellaria lateriflora	Nerve tonic, sedative, anti-spasmodic
Skunk cabbage	Encourages the elimination of toxins through the skin Anti-spasmodic and expectorant
Valerian Valeriana officinalis	Helps digestion and reduces gas Sedative, hypnotic, hypotensive and anti-spasmodic
Wild ginseng	Increases resistance and improves both physical and mental performance Sedative, anti-depressive and anti-spasmodic

It is important not to take too much of one particular herb because, after all, too much of anything can potentially do harm.

A few cups of herbal tea a day may be useful in severe cases. Use a combination of the herbs in each tea. You probably will find that the condition will improve as time goes by and you can cut down. Likewise, you can experiment with different combinations of the herbs to find the ones that suit you best. This list of effects that each herb may cause should help you to decide which ones are most suitable for you.

Case Studies

I have spoken to a few people who have been helped by herbal treatment. Sometimes the treatment has been more effective when taken as a longer term basis, and sometimes when taken on a short term basis - when the symptoms of a fit start occurring. I know of various people, husbands, wives, parents of epileptics etc who can see the symptoms of a fit coming on for maybe even a few days before it comes, whereas the epileptics themselves can't always tell the symptoms. In these cases it is possible to take the herbs sometime before the fit, without having to take them all the time.

Chapter 11 – Mind Control and Psychology

Introduction

There is definitely a certain amount of control that the mind can provide over the management of fits. This can vary considerably from person to person and can depend on the type of epilepsy, the volume and type of drugs taken and other factors. There are also some people, especially children and the mentally subnormal, who will bring on their seizures to gain attention or to get out of doing something that they don't want to do.

Rewards and Punishments

Some experimentation has been done by giving patients rewards for fit-free lengths of time or by punishing people for having fits. The use of rewards has helped, but it will only help certain people. After all, a long fit-free period for many people is a reward in itself and therefore any additional reward will make little difference. Punishing people for having fits is definitely not recommended.

Biofeedback

Biofeedback has been used with some success but is often rather impractical, mainly due to the expense involved. The patient is linked up to a machine that measures the various nerve impulses, as are measured in an EEG, and these are shown on the screen. The patient then tries to lower the stress level (or any other level that is being measured). This is done primarily through trial and error but because any changes made are shown on the screen, the patient can see what is happening and try to retain, or improve that state.

Hypnotherapy

This has had some success, especially in stress related conditions. It involves putting the patient in a light trance and using this to help them to remember various things that happened in the past that may be at the root of the stress related problems. This clears all the rubbish from the mind, fears based on childish views of the situation and so on, and helps the patient to adjust to life as it is, rather than worrying about unnecessary or imagined problems, which may be unconscious. Although this treatment can be rather expensive, it is something that only needs to be done once, usually over a period of about three months. Once completed it is no longer needed.

Some people worry about hypnotism, but there is no need to. You can certainly not be persuaded to do anything you do not want to, and all you really feel is being in a very relaxed state. However, some epileptics are advised against using hypnotherapy since it may trigger an attack, so it is important to speak to your practitioner about this. However, even if it does trigger an attack, it will not increase the number of fits in the long term and may well reduce them, and only you can decide whether you are willing to take this risk.

Treating Fits Preceded by Auras

Quite a lot of research has been done by Peter Fenwick and S.W. Brown on the treatment of fits that are preceded by auras. These are most suitable for psychological treatments because there is a period of time between noticing the aura and having the fit. In this time the person can use various techniques to stop the fit occuring. In time the aura may well disappear, or at least reduce in frequency and strength, as well as the fits.

The initial treatment in this is to relax the patient and then to get him to imagine the aura. From here he is asked to feel determined that he is not going to have a fit, so that the mental connection is made. This in itself should help to reduce the number of fits and, if the same procedure is used when the aura is felt, this should further reduce the chances.

In some cases, certain emotions will bring on a fit, such as fear or guilt. In this case the best course of action is to, where possible, eliminate these emotions. Since the emotions that bring on fits are usually especially severe, this is often possible without affecting the emotions felt in everyday life. The other procedure is to, in a similar way to that above, connect these emotions with relaxed feelings, so that the connection with the fit and the emotion is broken.

Focal Epilepsy

Focal epilepsy begins in one part of the body and then may spread into a complete fit. For instance, one finger may twitch or have a strange sensation in it, and the feeling will go up the arm and then through the whole body. The way to stop .this is to actively involve that finger in doing something else. This sounds very easy but is much more difficult than it sounds. However, it can be very successful.

Treating Yourself

If you come under any of the above categories you may be interested in trying the relevant procedures. If you do, be very careful and if you have any doubts, stop. The use of psychological treatments by the inexperienced, can do more harm than good. Have another look at Chapter 4, on Relaxation.

Chapter 12 – Bach Flower Remedies

Introduction

The Bach Flower Remedies aim to remove negative emotions and therefore improve the state of mind of the individual. Although this will not help epilepsy directly, it will help remove stress and other emotional factors so that you will feel better, and from here, it may lead to an improvement in all areas of health. The theory is that the flower remedies are in tune with higher frequencies of the mind and spirit.

Treatment with the Bach Flower Remedies aims to get to the root of your problems by treating one layer of emotions at a time. For each layer, a different remedy is required to handle the different emotions involved. In time, the treatment should get to the bottom layer and you should feel much better as you are not carrying around the subconscious emotional problems that you were before. During this process the symptoms may get worse for a while, but will then improve; worsening of the symptoms does show that the treatment is working.

The remedies are taken in the form of a few drops added to a drink or on the tongue two or three times a day. A combination of the different remedies may be taken, and the type of remedies will possibly be changed every month or so.

Treating Yourself

There is no specific qualification required to treat people with the Bach Flower Remedies, although many practitioners who are qualified in other areas will use this as well. This means that the treatment is not especially difficult. However it is useful to have someone objective around if you are treating yourself, since it is not always easy to be objective about your own emotions.

As with many other treatments, select those remedies from the list below which you think best suit your emotional state, a combination of up to six is usually used. Most of these remedies can be got in a health food shop, although addresses for obtaining are also found in Appendix 1. Follow the instructions on the bottle. After a month or so, review the situation and decide whether a change in remedies is required.

There are certain recommended combinations of remedies, the most useful one in the case of epilepsy is the Rescue Remedy that includes a combination of Star of Bethlehem, Rock Rose, Impatiens, Cherry Plum and Clematis. If possible, this should be given before a fit or during. If this is not possible then it should be taken immediately afterwards, and it will help the recovery. The Rescue Remedy is generally recommended for all cases of tension and shock.

The Remedies

Remedy	Negative State
Agrimony	Cheerful front covering mental torture
Aspen	Inexplicable fears and nightmares
Beech	Intolerance, criticism and arrogance
Centaury	Inability to refuse the demands of others
Cerato	Indecisiveness due to lack of confidence
Cherry Plum	Uncontrolled outbreaks of temper and fear of losing your mind
Chestnut Bud	Need for repetition and failure to learn by experience
Chicory	Possessiveness and self pity
Clematis	Little attention and indifference, daydreaming and unconsciousness
Crab Apple	Feeling of uncleanliness and self disgust, over emphasis on trivial details
Elm	Temporary and irrational feelings of inadequacy
Gentian	Easily discouraged
Gorse	Hopelessness and despair
Heather	Self centredness and a poor listener, fear of loneliness
Holly	Envy, jealousy, rage, suspicion or hatred
Honeysuckle	Homesickness and nostalgia
Hornbeam	Weariness

Impatiens	Impatience and irritability
Larch	Lack of confidence
Mimulus	Excessive fear of known things, such as dentist
Mustard	Periods of black depression
Oak	Despondency as the result of effort against all odds
Olive	Severe mental and physical exhaustion, particularly useful after a fit
Pine	Self reproach and guilt
Red Chestnut	Fear and excessive concern for the welfare of others
Rock Rose	Extreme fear, terror or panic
Rock Water	Too rigid self discipline, repression and self denial
Schleranthus	Indecision and uncertainty, mood swings
Star of Bethlehem	Mental and physical shock
Sweet Chestnut	Very extreme mental anguish
Vervain	Strain and tension as a result of over enthusiasm, hyperanxiety
Vine	Domineering and inflexible personality, always striving for power and ruthlessly ambitious
Walnut	Difficulty adjusting to change and oversensitivity to ideas and influences
Water Violet	Pride and aloofness
White Chestnut	Persistent worrying thoughts and mental arguments
Wild Oat	Dissatisfaction because your vocation hasn't been found, boredom and frustration
Wild Rose	Resignation and apathy
Willow	Bitterness and resentment, depression

Chapter 13 - Spiritual Healing

Introduction

Spiritual healing is something that many people will not even consider. They are a little frightened of it and are not really sure what to expect. Also, healing sometimes does get bad publicity. But there is nothing to be concerned about. Healers are no different to anyone else, you will find some who you like and some who you don't. In fact, probably you will find fewer healers who you don't like than you do members of the general public. There are also many different terms used for healing, and the way that the practitioner uses it may be different, but the basis of the treatment in all cases is very similar.

It is not necessary to be religious to take part in healing, it is not even necessary to believe that the treatment will work, although it will help. Although spectacular recoveries like you hear about do happen, it is more likely that there will be a gradual improvement of the condition. As with other complementary treatments, the peripheral symptoms often improve more than the fits. However repeated healing treatment will improve the condition.

The treatment usually involves sitting in a chair and relaxing whilst the healer places his hands on your head or shoulders. You are unlikely to feel anything beyond a sensation of warmth or pins and needles, and so there is very little to worry about. Occasionally a more violent reaction does occur but if it does it is a sign that your body is clearing out the toxins that are causing the problem.

It is difficult to give more information on this topic, since the treatment will vary from healer to healer and from client to client.

In acute cases it is often possible to perform healing at a distance, without actual contact being made between the healer and the patient.

Auras

One aspect of healing is the viewing of auras. Many healers can see these auras of varying colours which surround the body. The colours give some indication of the personality and health of the individual. In cases of epilepsy, these auras are often crooked and may have holes in them. Improvement in health can be achieved by the healer correcting these imbalances. These areas should not be confused with the auras felt before a fit, these are a completely different concept.

Treating Yourself

Although it is thought that most people have some degree of healing ability it can be limited, and also a certain amount of training and assistance is usually required. For this reason it is often not practical to treat yourself or to get a friend to treat you. However, no harm should come from reading around on the topic and experimenting a little yourself. There are also training courses on the topic available. However, many healers are cheap and will accept only a donation, especially if finances are low, so it may well be worth investigating if this interests you.

Case Studies

Alison was seven when she was first diagnosed as epileptic. When she was given conventional medication, although she was not having major seizures, she was having regular absences and periods when she was very dopey. She was then given spiritual healing. After the first two treatments she seemed to worsen a bit but after this she slowly improved. In time the drugs were slowly decreased. At the time of writing she has reached a plateau where she is on a minimum amount of the drugs, is not longer dopey and is having very few fits or absences. However, the treatment is still continuing.

Janet went into a grand mal seizure and then went into a coma. A group of healers tried distant healing on her, many of whom said that they saw an area of the brain that was discoloured. After this she noticeably improved.

Chapter 14 – Reflexology

Introduction

Reflexology is a treatment that stimulates or relaxes the body by the use of a massage of the feet. The theory is that all parts of the body are interconnected in many ways. One of these connections is that there is a link between each part of the body and a specific position on the foot. Massaging certain parts of the feet will encourage certain parts of the body to work better and therefore can improve many conditions. Tensions in certain parts of the body can be found by feeling certain parts of the feet.

The treatment is usually painless. If a part of the foot is pressed it is possible that there is short, sharp pain in a particular part of the body. This will point out where any problems exist and so will tell where treatment is needed.

Reflexology is particularly effective at treating back pain, insomnia, allergies, menstrual problems, migraine and asthma, so if you suffer from any of these it may well be worth a try. Also, many of these conditions have connections with epilepsy and I have heard of quite a few successes using this treatment.

Treating Yourself

Although it is impossible to treat yourself, due to the fact that you cannot relax and look at the soles of your feet at the same time, it is possible to get a friend to treat you. There are a variety of books available giving directions on how to treat with reflexology. Obviously some care is necessary since it is theoretically possible to trigger off a fit with reflexology. Although unlikely, if it does happen it may well be a sign of longer term improvement.

Be careful not to treat for too long at one time, since this can be exhausting and will become less effective. The first session may possibly last less than fifteen minutes although this can increase with time.

As always, a qualified therapist will be better and should be tried if at all possible.

Case Studies

Susan was 33 years old, she had bad circulation and brittle bones, but otherwise was in generally good health. She suffered from post-natal depression and epilepsy. She took anti-convulsants for three months during pregnancy. She had seven reflexology treatments and no fits occurred after the third treatment, and the depression lifted after six treatments.

She had no seizures until she was seven weeks pregnant. She then had nausea and many fits. At 18/19 weeks she was having three or four fits every night. She was hospitalised and given an intravenous glucose drip. Fits always occurred at night and the anticonvulsants did not help. She stopped taking the drugs in the last two months of pregnancy. She had a long labour that included a fit and gave birth to a baby girl. She had a fit on the third day. She started reflexology treatment when the baby was seven weeks old. There were one or two occasions when a fit seemed imminent but did not occur. There was a fit after the second treatment but with a quicker recovery than usual.

This epilepsy seemed to be induced by the pregnancy hormones. It may be that the frequency would have tailed off anyway until the second pregnancy, but the client felt more able to cope with the situation and did not take anticonvulsants during her second pregnancy, when the problem was far less anyway.

Julie, 26 years old – The following was written by her mother:

> Julie was born in Germany while her father was serving in the forces. At the time it was necessary for people to have the smallpox vaccination. The children were given it at about 13 months old along with the other immunisations.

94

Unfortunately Julie was the one in a million to react to it. She was left brain-damaged, though this was not apparent straight away.

Julie had been quite a smart young girl. At this young age she already had a vocabulary of about forty words and was learning fast. After this unfortunate happening the learning stopped. She had not forgotten anything but she was not taking anything new on board. Then she started falling down for no apparent reason. It was found that she had petit mal, one of the forms of epilepsy. By the time she was six years old she had the full blown grand mal as well as the petit mal form of epilepsy and was having to take drugs to control the fits.

Julie was taking: Zarontin capsules 1000 mg daily; Clobazam capsules 20 mg daily; Epanutin capsules 350 mg daily. It started with the Zarontin and gradually the others were introduced as they were necessary.

Julie's hearing and sight had been impaired along with the damage she had suffered. We had been told that the hearing and the sight would not get better, but with healing they have improved greatly. The fits were reasonably controlled, on average she would have a grand mal fit once in four or five weeks. Then about three years ago, while I was doing my training for the reflexology, the fits were coming each week and sometimes two within 24 hours.

As students of reflexology, we were told not to deal with such a case, but it was my daughter and I wished to do something to help her.

I started to give her a general treatment once a week. She had had a fit four days previous to the first treatment. I continued to give this treatment for four months. Then I would treat her maybe once a month. It was two years before she had another fit, and I feel this was because it had been three months since I had given her a treatment. It is now sometimes six weeks between treatments but she has gone another year now and has had no fits.

The treatment was of a general nature, giving no special attention to any part of the foot. Tenderness was noted in the areas of sinus, solar plexus, small intestine, liver and pancreas.

Chapter 15 – Acupuncture, Acupressure and Shiatsu

Introduction

Acupuncture and shiatsu are based on the same principles and the main difference is that acupuncture is done with the use of needles and shiatsu is done with the use of pressure.

The theory of acupuncture and shiatsu is that there are twelve meridians, or lines, on each side of the body, ten of which are connected to main organs. These contain vital energy, the strength of which depends on the state of the organ. The aim of the treatment is to stimulate this energy, in circumstances when the energy level is depleted, by the use of pressure or a needle in the relevant point.

Acupressure is slightly different in that it uses pressure to stimulate certain points rather than certain meridians.

The eastern concept of Yin/Yang – harmony and balance – is used. Yin and Yang are the two opposite sides of everything: hot and cold, dark and light and so on. However, most things will come somewhere in the middle and will not be all Yin or all Yang. The therapists try to balance out the Yin and Yang within the body.

A session will take from three quarters of an hour to an hour. The first one will begin with a discussion of medical history and other relevant details. Some analysis can be made just by looking at and listening to the patient.

Who Will it Help ?

The main uses of acupuncture and acupressure are to do the following:

- increase energy levels
- increase body awareness

- relieve stress related problems
- induce very deep relaxation
- ease aches and pains
- boost the immune system
- treat common ailments
- increase flexibility
- heal sports injuries
- stabilise emotional conditions
- relieve backache
- improve posture
- improve stamina
- improve digestion
- improve libido
- treat menstrual problems
- benefit healthy pregnancy
- ease childbirth
- relieve headaches and migraine

These treatments can be especially useful in conditions including allergies, stress and anxiety, and diabetes and hypoglycaemia, all of which can have an influence on epilepsy. Therefore, if the root of your problem lies in this area it may be worth trying. If your problem does not lie in these areas, or you are not sure, it may well be worth speaking to a local practitioner and seeing whether he or she thinks that they can help you.

Acupuncture

Many people are put off by the thought of acupuncture because they don't like the thought of having needles stuck into their bodies. Actually, it is usually completely painless. It is a treatment that has been used for many hundreds of years and therefore a fair amount of research has gone into it. Acupuncture is particularly useful in the areas of rheumatic problems, migraine and stress.

Acupressure and Shiatsu

Acupressure and shiatsu take the form of a massage, although somewhat different from the traditional type. It can be very invigorating and is very good for stress related problems. It involves the use of fingers, thumbs, palms, knees, forearms, elbows and feet. It is usually given on the floor with the patient wearing a single layer of cotton clothing.

Treating Yourself

Acupuncture should not be done by the inexperienced. The very basics of acupressure and shiatsu, however, can be learnt in a short time, although this is usually better done through a course rather than from a book. You cannot treat yourself by the use of shiatsu, so you will have to get a friend to treat you. Therefore I would suggest that if you want to try this, go to a qualified practitioner for one session and then decide if you would like to continue. You can learn the basic of acupressure, though, and treat minor conditions yourself. However, as always, an experienced and qualified practitioner will produce a greater effect.

Case Studies

Alison had brain damage and was having fits regularly. She was also very nervous, which caused her to have muscle spasms. In fact, she had to cancel her first two visits to the shiatsu practitioner because she was so nervous. However, when she began going regularly she noticed how much more relaxed she was and how she was generally better able to handle life. She had slightly fewer fits, and when she did have them she recovered much faster. She is still receiving treatment and is improving.

Martin was having one fit about every seven days. He went to see an acupuncturist. For the first two weeks his fits became more frequent and then he went for a period of six weeks without any. His condition has improved considerably, and he is now in the process of coming off his anticonvulsants.

Chapter 16 – Miscellaneous

Full Moon

One thing that has interested me in my research is the fact that fits tend to occur with the full moon. Unfortunately, to date, there seems to be no real solution to this problem, although many people are researching into various effects of the moon. The word epilepsy is actually derived from the Greek word for moon and there are many references to the relationship between the moon and fits, by early Latin and Greek authors.

Since menstruation also often occurs at the time of the full moon, it is not always easy in women to tell whether the fits occur in relation to the menstrual cycle or in relation to the moon. However, those women who are on the contraceptive pill will find that the moon and the menstrual cycle do not coincide, since the moon is on a 29 day cycle and menstruation will be on a 28 day cycle.

The Druids were great believers in the effect of the moon. They would harvest their mistletoe six days after the full moon and afterwards would sacrifice two white bulls and prepare a potion that was believed to act as a fertility drug for animals and women, an antidote for poison, a fire extinguisher and a cure for ulcers and epilepsy.

Other people believed that the reason that epilepsy and other conditions were more common at the full moon was due to demons whose activity depended on the phases of the moon. Similarly, in biblical times, it was believed that epilepsy was the effect of demons temporarily taking over the body as a punishment for having sinned, usually against the moon.

Other Cures

I received the following cures for epilepsy from the Gye Nyame

Spiritual Home in Ghana. I have not tried them, or spoken to anyone who has, but I expect that there must be a grain of truth in them.

• Take a turtle dove, cut its throat and let the patient drink its blood. He or she is free forever. Amen.

• Get some sea water, lagoon water, water from the lake or well, mix all together and read psalms 102, 109, 100 each once. Pronounce the holy name Elilahajah 80 times over it. Use it for drinking and for bathing. Amen, no more epilepsy by the grace of God.

• Get a fresh scaly fish, grind it and mix it with shea-butter, the bitter part of a cow (ox gall) and an egg. Repeat the above psalms and the holy names as instructed. Use the oil for rubbing and drinking a teaspoonful once a night. Amen. Jah Bless.

• Draw water from the stream around 5 am without speaking to anybody. Pick a frog from the stream and put it inside the bucketful of water drawn from the stream. Light a black consecrated candle and read from the Holy Bible Isaiah chapter 46. From the first verse to the end, into the water three times. Then bathe with it near the stream with a new sponge and soap which you have to throw away after the bath. After that take away the frog from the bucket, press its neck to force the mouth open, spit into its mouth and throw it from backward, looking back until you reach home.

Other Treatments

Below are listed a variety of alternative treatments, which may help to treat epilepsy. Contact names and books are listed in the Appendices.

ANTHROPOSOPHICAL MEDICINE

Anthroposophical medicine views the body as being in four parts, the physical, the astral, the etheric and the ego, and tries to get the correct balance between these. Treatment can include herbs, homoeopathy, massage, special baths, diet and art therapy. This treatment is especially useful for stress related conditions.

ART THERAPY

Art therapy involves expressing yourself through various forms of art such as painting and modelling. This therapy aims at getting to the root of your emotions and can be very enjoyable, it is especially useful for children since they do not feel like they are being treated and therefore are more relaxed.

ASTROLOGICAL COUNSELLING

Astrological counselling is a form of counselling which involves using the birth details and the positions of the planets throughout the person's life. This helps to understand the psychological influences which have happened throughout the lifetime and therefore to get to the root of the problems.

AYURVEDA

Ayurveda works on the basis that most people are primarily one of three types. They are either air and space, earth and water, or fire. Many other factors are also taken into consideration. Treatment is in the form of gems, metal, herbs and oils.

BIODYNAMICS

Biodynamics works on the basis that the digestive system holds the clues to our health. It is done by listening to the stomach and then treating it by massage. It is particularly good for stress related conditions.

BIOENERGETICS

The aim of bioenergetics is to integrate the body and the emotions. It works by using a series of exercises. This is particularly useful for stress related conditions.

BIOLOGICAL MEDICINE

Biological medicine believes in the necessity for eliminating toxic waste from the body. Diagnosis is done by the use of Voll and Vega machines. Treatment is done with herbs, homoeopathy and acupuncture. Since the build up of toxins is often a feature of epilepsy this could be very helpful.

COLONIC IRRIGATION

Colonic irrigation can come under various other similar names. It works on the basis that the colon holds a great many toxins that must be eliminated from the body. Although it sounds uncomfortable it can actually be quite enjoyable. It involves injecting water through the anus and then releasing it again. I have heard of some success in treating epilepsy with this method.

COLOUR THERAPY

Colour therapy is based on the fact that colour can have a great influence on us. Therefore colour can be used to adjust any imbalances that we may have in our bodies, minds or spirits. Colour therapy can be used in all types of conditions.

CRYSTAL HEALING

Many people have gained noticeable improvements, if not complete cures, from crystal healing. There is a growing following in the use of crystals for healing and relaxation prevention of certain illnesses. Crystals can produce electro-magnetic energy which can be put to many uses. It is a vitalising force that will stimulate the energy levels of all individuals who happen to be near to the crystal. This will lead to a spiritual quickening and a raising of levels of consciousness. All crystals absorb the energies present during their growth period into their structure, and output these later.

The use of crystals involves energising the crystals to ensure that you get full value of their powers. These powers can be directed in certain directions, whether healing, relaxation or whatever else is required. Different crystals have different powers. Jasper is the one that is used to treat epilepsy.

DANCE THERAPY

Dance helps release the individual from both physical and emotional stress. It also helps to keep the body fit. There are many different ways in which it can be used, in groups or individually, and many different types of dancing. Dance therapy can help people to express themselves who may not find it easy to talk about their feelings.

DOWSING

Dowsing is a form of diagnosis. It involves using a pendulum to pick up energy vibrations and imbalances. From this diagnosis, recommendations can be made.

DREAM THERAPY

Dream therapy involves the analysis of your dreams to get to the root of your emotional, and maybe physical problems. You write your dreams down every day and the therapist analyses the main aspects of these to find the common threads.

HELLERWORK

Hellerwork uses physical exercise to release memory of traumatic experiences, therefore to bring stress to the surface and to release it.

IRIDOLOGY

Iridology is a form of diagnosis that uses the iris of the eye. Parts of the body are related to parts of the iris, and the practitioner can help get to the root of your problem or see potential problems, which may otherwise go unnoticed until they become more serious.

KINESIOLOGY

Kinesiology involves using a series of muscle tests to measure the energy flow and to find where problems arise. It can also be used to treat these problems. It can be particularly useful in stress related problems.

MEDIUMSHIP

This can be another form of diagnosis. A medium may be able to give advice on how to sort out your problems, including health ones.

METAMORPHIC TECHNIQUE

The Metamorphic technique aims to access the individual's innate intelligence and use this to find a cure for the problems. This is done by lightly touching the spinal reflex points on the feet, hands and head.

MUSIC THERAPY

Music therapy is similar, in a way, to dance therapy. It helps people to express themselves without having to do it verbally. Although some talking is involved, music is used to help change the mood and relax the patient.

OLIGO-ELEMENTS

Oligo-elements are metals or metalloids which cannot be produced by the human being but can be found in plants as trace elements. These metals are required to adjust the chemical processes in our body which ensure the proper operation of the organs. These elements are used in liquid form in naturopathy and homoeopathy. Boron and bromine can be used to help epilepsy and a vanadium-lithium combination helps in neuropsychological conditions. Various different applications of this process are used in other forms of treatment.

POLARITY THERAPY

Polarity therapy involves the patient lying down and being gently pressed in certain areas by the therapist. This enables them to find the problems in the energy flow and then to help correct any imbalances that are present.

REBIRTHING

Rebirthing is a form of regression which enables the patient to relive their birth and the traumas which went with it. This then releases any psychological influences of the trauma and should help stress related problems. If your epilepsy started when you were fairly young and is stress related, this may help.

REGRESSION THERAPY

Regression therapy involves using a light hypnotic trance to regress the patients to previous lives. The therapists believe that there are many traumas in past lives that reflect upon present lives, and the acceptance of these traumas will help the patient to come to terms with present problems. Practitioners say that they usually cannot prove these past lives, but the treatment can help many mental and physical problems.

TIBETAN PULSING

Tibetan pulsing releases trapped energy by stimulating pulse beats that can be felt around the body.

Appendix 1 Addresses

Chapter 1 – Allergies

Action Against Allergy

43 The Downs, London SW20 8HG

A support group for allergy sufferers, providing a regular newsletter.

British Society for Clinical Ecology

Burgh Wood Clinic, 34 Brighton Road, Banstead, Surrey SM7 1BS

Royal Liverpool Hospital, Prescot Street, Liverpool, L7 8XP.

Aims to widen understanding of clinical ecology and allergy related problems.

Chapman and Smith Ltd.

Safin Works, East Hoathly, nr. Lewes, BN8 6EW

Produce masks which protect against fumes and chemicals.

Foodwatch International Ltd.

9 Corporation Street, Taunton, Somerset TA1 4AJ

☎ 0823 325022

Provide Vega allergy and vitamin deficiency tests throughout England.

Cow and Gate Ltd.

Trowbridge, Wiltshire

Produce soya protein infant formula foods.

Environmental Medicine Foundation

Symondsbury House, Bridport, Dorset DT6 6HB

Environmental Paints Ltd.

Unit 11, Dunscar Industrial Estate, Blackburn Road, Egerton, Bolton BL7 9PQ

☎ 0204 596854

Produce non toxic paints.

Food Watch

High Acre, East Stour, Gillingham, Dorset, SP8 5JR

Mail Order service supplying additive free foodstuffs.

The Healthy House

Cold Harbour, Ruscombe, Stroud, GL6 4DA

☎ 0453 752216

Provide a range of allergy free products.

Henry Doubleday Research Association

Ryton on Dunsmore, Coventry, CV8 3LG

Advises on all aspects of non-chemical agriculture.

Holistic Health Centre

85 Dunnings Road, East Grinstead, West Sussex, RH19 4AQ

☎ 0342 323120

Provide Vega allergy tests.

Human Ecology Research Foundation of the South West Inc.

12110 Webbs Chapel Road, Suite E-305, Dallas, Texas 75234, USA

Produce a cotton face mask with a charcoal filter to minimise the effects of traffic fumes.

Institute of Allergy Therapists

Ffynnonwen, Llangwyryfon, Aberyswyth, Dyfed

☎ 09747 376

Has a register of trained practitioners.

Larkhall Laboratories

225 Putney Bridge Road, London SW15

Supplies mail order gluten free flours and other food substitutes.

Livos Natural Paint Products

PO Box 103, Warwick CV34 6QZ

☎ 0926 400821

Supply non toxic paint.

Moulinex

Station Approach, Coulsdon, Surrey

Manufacture a small mill which can grind substitutes into flour.

National Society for Research into Allergy

PO Box 50, Hinckley, Leicestershire, LE10 1JY

Primrose Healing Centre

9 St George's Mews, Primrose Hill, London NW1 8XE

☎ 071 586 0148

Real Foods Ltd

37 Broughton Street, Edinburgh EH1 3JU

Natural and organic foods delivered to the door.

Shakless International Health Foods

15 Cotteridge Close, Stony Stratford, Milton Keynes

Supply a range of concentrated organic cleaners.

Society for Environmental Therapy

3 Atherton Road, Ipswich, Suffolk IP4 2LD

Discusses the environmental causes of disease, publishes a regular newsletter.

Society of Alternative Therapists
15 Station Road, Sidcup, Kent DA15 7EN
☎ 081 300 3348
Provide Vega allergy testing.

Soil Association
86-88 Colston Street, Bristol, BS1 5BB
Advises on all aspects of non-chemical agriculture.

Wyeth Laboratories
Taplow, Maidenhead, Berkshire
Produce soya protein infant formula foods.

Chapter 2 – Vitamins and Minerals

British Nutrition Foundation
15 Belgrave Square, London SW1X 8PS
☎ 071 235 4904

British Society for Nutritional Medicine
PO Box 3AP, London W1A 3AP
Aims to widen the understanding of the role of nutrition in health and illness and to encourage relevant research.

C. Thomas
46 Caistor Park Road, Stratford, London E15 3PT
Nutritional therapist with experience of epilepsy.

Green Farm
Burwash Common, East Sussex TN19 7LX
☎ 0435 882482
Nutritional Therapy.

Institute of Optimum Nutrition

5 Jerdan Place, London SW6 1BE

☎ 071 385 7984

McCarrison Society

24 Paddington Street, London W1M 4DR.

Society for the Promotion of Nutritional Medicine

2 Hampden Lodge, Hailsham Road, Heathfield, East Sussex TN21 8AE

☎ 0435 867007

Chapter 3 – Hormones

The National Association for Pre-menstrual Syndrome

PO Box 72, Sevenoaks, Kent TN13 1XQ

Chapter 4 – Relaxation

British Tai Chi Association

7 Upper Wimpole Street, Marylebone, London, W1M 7TD

☎ 071 935 8444

British Wheel of Yoga

1 Hamilton Place, Boston Road, Sleaford, Lincolnshire, NG34 7ES

☎ 0529 306851

Float Centre

20 Blenheim Terrace, St Johns Wood, London NW8 0EB

☎ 071 328 7276

Floatation Tank Association

3A Elms Crescent, London SW4

Iyengar Yoga Institute

223a Randolph Avenue, London W9 1NL

☎ 071 624 3080

London and Counties Society of Physiologists

100 Waterloo Road, Blackpool, Lancashire FY4 1AW

☎ 0253 403548

London College of Massage

5 Newman Passage, London W1P 3PF

☎ 071 323 3574

New World Cassettes

Paradise Farm, Westhall, Halesworth, Suffolk, IP19 8RH

Provide a range of relaxation and other tapes.

Relaxation for Living

29 Burwood Park Road, Walton-on-Thames, Surrey KT12 5LH

☎ 0932 227826

Provide a list of relaxation teachers, books, tapes etc.

School of Meditation

158 Holland Park Avenue, London W11 4UH

☎ 071 603 6116

School of Tai Chi Chuan

Centre for Healing, 5 Tavistock Place, St Pancras, London WC1 9HH

☎ 081 459 0764

Sivananda Yoga Centre

51 Felsham Road, London SW15

☎ 081 780 0160

Transcendental Meditation
24 Linhope Street, Marylebone, London NW1 6TH
☎ 071 402 3452

Transcendental Meditation National Office
Mentmore Towers, Mentmore, Leighton Buzzard LU7 0QH

Yoga for Health Foundation
Ickwell Bury, Northill, Biggleswade, Bedfordshire SG18 9EF
☎ 076 727 271
Hold a variety of residential programmes for the sick and the healthy in very relaxed surroundings and at very realistic prices.

Chapter 5 – Chiropractice, Osteopathy and Cranial Massage

British and European Osteopathic Association
6 Adelaide Road, Teddington, Middlesex TW11 0AY

British Chiropractic Association
Premier House, 10 Greycoat Place, London SW1P 1SB
☎ 071 222 8866

College of Osteopaths Practitioners Association
1 Furzehill Road, Borehamwood, Herts WD6 2DG
☎ 081 905 1937

The Cranial Osteopathic Association
478 Baker Street, Enfield, Middx, EN1 3QS
☎ 081 367 5561

Craniosacral Therapy Educational Trust

29 Dollis Park, Finchley Central, London N3 1HJ

☎ 081 349 0297

General Council and Register of Osteopaths

☎ 0734 576585

The Institute of Pure Chiropractic

14 Park End Street, Oxford OX1 1HH

☎ 0865 246687

Natural Therapeutic and Osteopathic Society

14 Marford Road, Wheathampstead, Herts AL4 8AS

☎ 0582 833950

Chapter 6 – Low Blood Sugar

The Bournemouth Complementary Medical Practice

3 Lorne Park Road, Bouremouth BH1 1LD

Produce a list of people who can test patient for hypoglycaemia with the six hour glucose tolerance test.

Chapter 7 – Detoxification

J G Levenson

1 Welbeck House, 62 Welbeck Street, London W1M 7HB

☎ 071 486 3127

Provides list of holistic dentists and tests for mercury poisoning.

Chapter 8 – Aromatherapy

Aromatherapy Quarterly

Dept T, 5 Ranelagh Avenue, London SW13 0BY

The longest running English language magazine in the aromatherapy world.

The Astral Beauty Institute, Bournemouth

☎ 0202 318267

New Age Aromatherapy – combining essential oils with healing.

International Federation of Aromatherapists

Department of Continuing Education, Royal Masonic Hospital, Ravenscourt Park, London W6 0TN

☎ 081 846 8066

International Society of Professional Aromatherapists

41 Leicester Road, Hinckley, LE10 1LW

☎ 0455 637987

The Register of Qualified Aromatherapists

26 Roden Court, Hornsey Lane, London N6 5NN

Tisserand Association for Holistic Aromatherapists

65 Church Road, Hove, East Sussex, BN3 2BD

☎ 0273 206640

Chapter 9 – Homoeopathy

Ainsworths Homoeopathic Pharmacy

38 New Cavendish Street, London, W1M 7LH

Orders: 40-44 High Street, Caterham, Surrey, CR3 5UB

☎ 0883 340332

Fax: 0883 344602

British Homoeopathic Association

27A Devonshire Street, London W1N 1RJ

☎ 071 935 2163

Aims to promote homoeopathy, produces a bimonthly newsletter, has a lending library and provides, advice, lectures, etc.

Hahnemann Society

Hahnemann House, 2 Powis Place, Great Ormond Street, London WC1N 3HT

Campaign for homoeopathy's rights in the NHS, produce regular magazine.

Homoeopathic Development Foundation

19a Cavendish Square, London W1M 9AD

Nelsons Homoeopathic Pharmacy

73 Duke Street, Grosvenor Square, London, W1M 6BY

☎ 071 629 3118

Society of Homoeopaths

Artizan Road, Northampton NN1 4HU

☎ 0604 21400

UK Homoeopathic Medical Association

243 The Broadway, Southall, Middlesex, UB1 1NF

☎ 081 843 9220/081 577 7781

Fax: 081 843 9220

Professional body of UK homoeopaths.

Chapter 10 – Herbal Treatment

British Herbal Medicine Association

Field House, Lye Hole Lane, Redhill, Avon BS18 7TB

☎ 0934 862994

General Council and Register of Consultant Herbalists

Grosvenor House, 40 Seaway, Middleton-on-Sea, West Sussex PO22 7SA

☎ 0243 586012

National School of Herbal Medicine

Bucksteep Manor, Bodle Street Green, Hailsham, East Sussex BN27 4RJ

☎ 0323 833812

National Institute of Medical Herbalists

9 Palace Gate, Exeter, Devon EX1 1JA

☎ 0392 426022

Chapter 11 – Mind Control and Psychology

Academy and Professional Hypnotherapy Association

181 Cat Hill, Cockfosters, East Barnet, Herts EN4 8HS

☎ 081 441 9685

Acumedic Centre

101-103 Camden High Street, Camden, London NW1

☎ 071 388 5783, 071 388 6704

The Adlerian Society

55 Mayhill Road, London SE7 7JG

☎ 081 858 7299

Association for Humanistic Psychology

26 Huddlestone Road, London E7 0AN

☎ 081 555 3077

Association of Humanistic Psychology Practitioners

87 Whipps Cross Road, Leytonstone, London E11 1NJ

☎ 081 455 8737/081 530 3283

Association of Jungian Analysts
3-7 Eton Avenue, South Hampstead, London NW3
☎ 071 794 8711

Astro-Psychotherapeutic Practice
1 Grafton Road, Acton, London W3 6PB
☎ 081 992 9514

Audio Limited
26-28 Wendell Road, London W12
☎ 081 743 1518 or 081 743 4352

Bexleyheath Natural Health Clinic
6 Sandford Road, Bexleyheath, Kent DA7 4AX
☎ 081 303 9571

British Association for Counselling
37A Sheep Street, Rugby CV21 3BX
☎ 0788 578328

British Association for the Person-Centred Approach
London WC1N 3XX

British Association of Psychotherapists
121 Hendon Lane, Hendon, London N3 3PR
☎ 081 346 1747

British Hypnosis Research
8 Paston Place, Brighton BN2 1HA
☎ 0273 693622

British Hypnotherapy Centre
1 Wythburn Place, London W1H 5WL
☎ 071 262 8852

British Psycho-Analytical Society
63 New Cavendish Street, London W1
☎ 071 636 2322

Brunel Management Programme
Brunel University, Uxbridge, Middlesex UB8 3PH
☎ 0895 56461 x 215

Centre for Alternative Education and Research
Rosemerryn, Lamorna, Penzance, Cornwall TR19 6BN
☎ 0736 810530

Centre for Counselling and Psychotherapy Education
21 Lancaster Road, London W11 1QL
☎ 071 221 3215

Centre for Stress Management
☎ 081 293 4114

Chessington Hypnotherapy Clinic
130 Guilders Road, Chessington, Surrey
☎ 081 397 3146

Communication and Counselling Foundation
Haflodas, Tregoran, Dyfed, Wales SY25 6UG
☎ 0974 298998/0570 570831

Corporation of Advanced Hypnotherapy
PO Box 70, Southport, PR9 9HR

Equilibrium Therapy Centre
117 Granville Road, Southfields, London SW18 5SF
☎ 081 870 8761

Gestalt Centre London
64 Warwick Road, St Albans, Herts AL1 4DL
☎ 0727 64806

Gestalt Therapy in West London
36 Newburgh Road, Acton, London W3 6DQ
☎ 081 993 0868

Holwell Centre for Psychodrama and Sociodrama
East Down, Barnstaple, Devon EX31 3NZ
☎ 0271 850267 / 0271 850597

Human Potential Resource Group
Department of Educational Studies, University of Surrey, Guildford,
Surrey GU2 5XH
☎ 0483 509191

The Institute for the Arts in Psychotherapy
1 Beaconsfield Road, St Albans, Herts AL1 3RD
☎ 0438 833440

The Institute for Traditional and Humanistic Psychotherapy
☎ 081 995 7175

International Association of Hypno-Analysts
PO Box, 180, Bournemouth, Dorset BH3 7AD
☎ 0202 304624

International Psychoanalytic Association

Broomhills, Woodside Lane, London N12

☎ 081 446 8324

London Society for Ericksonian Psychotherapy and Hypnosis

1 Mill Lane, Stedham, Midhurst, West Sussex GU29 0RS

☎ 083 081 5613

Medical and Dental Hypnosis Society

The Practice, 24 Skye Crescent, Paisley PA2 8EL.

☎ 0698 854048

National Council of Psychotherapists and Hypnotherapy Register

46 Oxhey Road, Oxhey, Watford, Herts WD1 4QQ

☎ 0923 227772

National Register of Hypnotherapists and Psychotherapists

12 Cross Street, Nelson, Lancs BB9 7EN

☎ 0282 699378

Natureworks

16 Balderton Street, London W1

☎ 071 355 4036

Neal's Yard Therapy Rooms

2 Neal's Yard, Covent Garden, London WC2

☎ 071 379 7662

Psychosynthesis and Education Trust

48 Guildford Road, Stockwell, London SW8 2BU

☎ 071 633 8295

Skills with People

15 Liberia Road, Islington, London N5 1JP

☎ 071 359 2370/071 368 3605

Society of Analytical Psychology

1 Daleham Gardens, Swiss Cottage, London NW3 5BY

☎ 071 435 7696

Women's Therapy Link

☎ 081 442 4998

Provide psychotherapy and counselling for women in practices throughout London.

Chapter 12 – Bach Flower Remedies

The Bach Centre

Mount Vernon, Sotwell, Wallingford, Oxfordshire, OX10 0PZ

☎ 0491 39489/34678

The Flower Remedy Programme

PO Box 65, Hereford, HR2 0UW

Chapter 13 – Spiritual Healing

Association for Therapeutic Healers

Flat 5, 54-56 Neal Street, Covent Garden, London WC2

☎ 071 240 0176

Laurence Dayan

☎ 071 381 4729

Healer with experience of epilepsy.

Matthew Manning Centre

Buryfields, Cage End, Hatfield Broad Oak, Bishops Stortford, Herts CM22 7HT

☎ 0279 70330

National Federation of Spiritual Healers

Old Manor Farm Studio, Church Street, Sunbury-on-Thames, Middlesex TW16 6RG

☎ 0932 783164

Chapter 14 – Reflexology

Association of Reflexologists

110 John Silkin Lane, London SE8 5BE

☎ 071 237 6523

British Reflexology Association

Monks Orchard, Whitbourne, Worcs, WR6 5RB

☎ 0886 21207

Kristine Walker

40 Stanmer Villas, Brighton, E Sussex BN1 7HP

☎ 0273 508398 (after 4pm)

Reflexologist with experience of treating epilepsy.

Margaret England

9 Tallis Grove, Inns Court, Knowle, Bristol BS4 1XB

Reflexologist with experience of treating epilepsy.

☎ 0272 782743

Reflexologists' Society

39 Prestbury Road, Cheltenham, Glos, GL52 2PT

☎ 0242 512601

Wholistic Association of British Reflexologists

92 Sheering Road, Old Harlow, Essex CM17 0JW

☎ 0279 429060

Chapter 15 – Acupuncture, Acupressure and Shiatsu

Academy of Chinese Acupuncutre

15-17 Southend Road, London NW3

☎ 071 794 0848

Andy Harrop

☎ 081 299 2152

Shiatsu practitioner with experience in epilepsy.

British Acupuncture Association

Alderney Street, London SW1V 4EU

☎ 071 834 1012 / 071 834 6229

The Register of Traditional Chinese Medicine

19 Trinity Road, London N2 8JJ

☎ 081 883 8431

Publishes an annual list of qualified acupuncture practitioners.

The Shiatsu Society

14 Oakdene Road, Redhill, Surrey RH1 6BT

☎ 0737 767896

Traditional Acupuncture Society

1 The Ridgeway, Stratford Upon Avon, Warwickshire CV3ʳ

Chapter 16 – Miscellaneous

ANTHROPOSOPHICAL MEDICINE

Anthroposophical Medicine

Rudolph Steiner House, 35 Park Road, London NW1 6XT

☎ 071 723 4400

ART THERAPY

Art from Within

119 Grosvenor Avenue, Highbury, London N5 2NL

☎ 071 354 1603

British Association of Art Therapists Ltd.

11a Richmond Road, Brighton BN2 3RL

Creative Arts Workshops

Margot Sutherland, Terpsichore, 70 Cranwich Road, London N16 5JD

☎ 081 809 5866

Institute of Arts in Therapy and Education

70 Cranwich Road, N16 5JD

☎ 081 809 5866

Living Art

11 Stowe Road, London W12 8BQ

☎ 081 749 0874

Art Therapy.

Person-Centred Art Therapy Centre

1 Cranbourne Gardens, London NW11 0HN

☎ 081 455 8570

Playspace
Short Course Unit, University of Westminster, 35 Marylebone Road,
Marylebone, London NW1 5LS
☎ 071 486 5811 x 465

Astro-Psychotherapeutic Practice
1 Grafton Road, Acton, London W3 6PB
☎ 081 992 9514

Centre for Psychological Astrology
PO Box 890, London NW3 2JZ
☎ 071 223 2478

Cheirological Society
18 Southerton Road, Hammersmith, London W6

AYURVEDA

Maharishi Ayurveda Health Centre
20 Wimpole Street, London W1M 7AD
☎ 071 436 4583

Maharishi Ayurveda Health Centre
Woodley Park Road, Skelmersdale, Lancs WN8 6UQ
☎ 0695 51008

BIODYNAMICS

Gerda Boyesen Institute
120 The Vale, London W3 7RQ
☎ 081 746 0499
Bioenergetics.

Association of Biodynamic Psychotherapists
153 Goldhurst Terrace, London NW6 3EU.
☎ 071 328 3868

Bioenergetic Training Association for Great Britain
22 Fitzjohn's Avenue, Swiss Cottage, London NW3
☎ 071 435 1079

Human Potential Resource Group
Department of Educational Studies, University of Surrey, Guildford,
Surrey GU2 5XH
☎ 0483 509191

Maitri
Little Abshott Road, Titchfield, Hants PO14 4LN
☎ 0489 572451

BIOLOGICAL MEDICINE

Society of Biological Medicine
398 Uxbridge Road, Hatch End, Pinner, Middlesex HA5 4HP
☎ 081 428 4333
Biological Medicine.

COLONIC IRRIGATION

Colonic International Association
50A Morrish Road, London SW2 4EG
☎ 081 671 7136

International Colon Hydrotherapy Foundation
27 Warwick Avenue, London W9 2PS
☎ 071 289 7000

COLOUR THERAPY

International Association for Colour Healers
Endellion, Money Row Green, Holyport, Maidenhead, Berkshire SL6 2HA
☎ 0628 34777

International Association of Colour Therapists
Brook House, Avening, Tetbury, Gloucestershire GL8 8NS
☎ 045383 2150

CRYSTAL HEALING

Crystal 2000
37 Bromley Road, St Annes on Sea, Lancs FY8 1PQ
☎ 0253 723735

International Association of Crystal Healing Therapists
5 Sunnymede Vale, Holcombe Brook, Bury, Lancs BL0 9RR
☎ 020488 3482

The School of Electro-crystal Therapy
117 Long Drive, South Ruislip, Middlesex, HA4 0HL
☎ 081 841 1716

DANCE THERAPY

5 to Midnight
5 Bittaford Terrace, Bittaford, South Devon, PL21 0DX
☎ 0752 894675

Association for Dance Movement Therapy
99 South Hill Park, Hampstead NW3 2SP
☎ 071 794 9833

Creative Arts and Therapy Consultants

Margot Sunderland, Terpsichore, 70 Cranwich Road, London N16 5JD

☎ 081 809 5866

Dancing on the Path

39A Glengarry Road, London SE22

☎ 081 693 6953

DOWSING

British Society of Dowsers

Sycamore Cottage, Hastingleigh, Ashford, Kent TN25 5HW

☎ 0233 75253

Jack Temple

Bluegate Nursery House, Pyrford Road, Pyrford, Woking, Surrey GU22 8UQ

☎ 0932 342429

Runs courses on dowsing.

DREAM THERAPY

Abraxas

27 Bathurst Mews, London W2 2SB

☎ 071 402 0290

Imprint

377 Wimbledon Park Road, London SW19 6PE

☎ 081 788 1500

IRIDOLOGY

National Council and Register of Iridologists

40 Stokewood Road, Bournemouth, BH3 7NE

☎ 0202 529793

KINESIOLOGY

Association for Systematic Kinesiology
39 Browns Road, Surbiton, Surrey KT5B 8ST

Kinesiology for Health and Wellbeing
39 Browns Road, Surbiton, Surrey KT5 8ST

MEDIUMSHIP

College of Psychic Studies
16 Queensberry Place, London SW7 2EB
☎ 071 589 3292/3

METAMORPHIC TECHNIQUE.

The Metamorphic Association
67 Ritherdon Road, Tooting, London SW17 8QE
☎ / Fax: 081 672 5951

MUSIC THERAPY

Mu Sum Ba
93 Percy Road, London W12 9QH
☎ 081 743 7246

Nordoff-Robbins Music Therapy Centre
6 Queensdale Walk, London W12 4QQ

OLIGO-ELEMENTS

Herbamin Arophar UK
PO Box 5, Albury, Surrey, GU5 9DN
☎ 048641 2047
Arophar Micro Element Bio-Catalytic Cellular stockist.

POLARITY THERAPY

Polarity Therapy Association UK
11 Willow Vale, Frome, Somerset BA1 11BG
☎ 0373 452250

REBIRTHING

Centre for Alternative Education and Research
Rosemerryn, Lamorna, Penzance, Cornwall TR19 6BN
☎ 0736 810530

Rebirthing Centre
Flat B, 2 Wandsworth Common West Side, Wandsworth, London
SW18 2EL
☎ 081 870 9284

REGRESSION THERAPY

British Foundation Past Life Therapy/Research
081 505 8720

Denise Linn, Lisha Simester
☎ 071 938 3788
Run workshops and training seminars.

Dr Roger Woolger
☎ 0867 307996
Runs workshops and training seminars.

Ros Bamkin
☎ 081 902 5253
Individual sessions and group classes.

OTHER

Association of General Practitioners of Natural Medicine
38 Nigel House, Portpool Lane, London EC1N 7UR
☎ 071 405 2781

British Complementary Medicine Association
St Charles Hospital, Exmoor Street, London W10 6DZ
☎ 081 964 1205

British Holistic Medical Association
179 Gloucester Place, London NW1 6DX
Aims to encourage holistic medicine.

City Health Centre
36-37 Featherstone Street, London EC1Y 8QX
☎ 071 251 4429
A clinic providing a range of alternative therapies.

Community Health Foundation
188 Old Street, London EC1V 9BP
☎ 071 251 4076
Hold a wide range of courses in many areas of alternative medicine.

Council for Complementary and Alternative Medicine
179 Gloucester Place, London, NW1 6DX
☎ 071 724 9103

Cygmus Book Club
PO Box 147, Redhill, Surrey RH1 6FH
Book club on mind, body and spirit matters.

Dr Ian MacDonald

Rectory Lodge, Church Green, Ovingdean, East Sussex BN2 7BA

☎ 0273 307537

An osteopath, naturopath and homoeopath with experience of treating epilepsy.

General Council and Register of Naturopaths

6 Netherhall Gardens, London, NW3 5RR

☎ 071 435 8728

The Greenhouse

Bangor, Gwynedd, LL57 1AX

☎ 0248 355821

Offers a variety of alternative treatments.

Hilary Davidson

521 Foxhall Road, Ipswich, Suffolk IP3 8LW

☎ 0473 723552

An acupuncturist and nutritional therapist with experience of treating epilepsy.

Holistic Emporium

Hyden House Ltd, Little Hyden Lane, Clanfield, Hants, PO8 0RU

☎ 0705 596500

Fax: 0705 596500

Sell a wide range of natural medicines.

Holistic Health Concessions Register

36 Broadway Market, Hackney, London E8 4QJ

☎ 071 254 1158

Incorporated Society of Registered Naturopaths

1 Albemarle Road, The Mount, York YO2 1EN

Institute of Complementary Medicine

PO Box 194, London SE16 1QZ

☎ 071 237 5165

International Register of Oriental Medicine

Green Hedges House, Green hedges Avenue, East Grinstead, Sussex RH19 1DZ

☎ 0342 313106/7

The Nutri Centre

7 Park Crescent, London W1N 3HE

☎ 071 436 5122/071 631 0156

Have a wide range of vitamins and minerals, homoeopathic treatments, aromatherapy supplies and so on. Will provide mail order service.

Pilgrim Books

48 Culver Street, Newent, Glos. GL18 1DA

☎ 0531 821075

The Radionics Association

Baerlein House, Goose Green, Deddington, Oxford OX15 4SZ

☎ 0869 38852

Sanity

63 Cole Park Road, Twickenham, Middlesex, TW1 1HT

Collects information on nutritional and environmental factors in mental illness.

Appendix 2 Further Reading

Chapter 1 – Allergies

Against the Unsuspected Enemy, Amelia Nathan-Hill, New Horizon, 1980

Allergies, your Hidden Enemy, Theron G Randolph and Ralph W Moss, Turnstone Press, 1981

Allergy and Intolerance – A Complete Guide to Environmental Medicine, George Lewith, Julian Kenyon and David Dowson, Merlin Press, London

The Allergy Diet, Workman, Jones and Hunter, Addenbrookes Hospital, Dunitz

Allergy Prevention for Kids, Dr Leo Galland

The Allergy Problem Vicky Reppere, Thorsons 1983

Clinical Ecology, Edited by Lawrence D Dickey, Charles C Thomas, 1976

Collins Gem Guide to Natural and Artificial Food Additives, John Clark, Harper Collins

The Complete Wheat Free Cookbook, Dr Sheila Gibson, Louise Templeton and Dr Robin Gibson, Thorsons

Cooking Without, Barbara Cousins, Moorside Natural Healing Clinic. Recipes free of wheat, sugar, dairy foods, fat, salt and yeast.

Detecting Your Hidden Allergies, William Crook.

Dr Atkins' Nutrition Breakthrough, Robert C Atkins, Bantam/Perigord 1981.

Easy Vegetarian Cookery, David Eno, Thorsons.

Eating and Allergy, Robert Eagle, Thorsons, 1986.

E for Additives, Maurice Hanssen, Thorsons, 1984.

Encyclopedia of Allergy and Environmental Illness – A Self Help Approach, Ellen Rothera, David and Charles, Newton Abbot

The Food Allergy Plan, Keith Mumby

The Food Watch Alternative Cookbook, Honor J Campbell, Ashgrove Press Ltd.

The Gluten Free and Wheat Free Bumper Bake Book, Rita Greer, Bluebird Ltd

The Gluten Free Diet Book, Dr Peter Rawcliffe and Ruth Rolph, Macdonald Optima

Health on your Plate , Janet Pleshette, Hamlyn Paperbacks, 1983

How to Eat Well Again on a Wheat, Gluten and Dairy Free Diet, Fran Crosthwaite, Diet Care

The New E for Additives, Maurice Hanssen with Jill Marsden, Thorsons

The Organic Food Guide, Edited by Alan Gear, Henry Doubleday Research Association, 1983

Orthomolecular Nutrition, A Hoffer, Keats 1978

Provocative Testing and Injection Therapy, Joseph B Miller, Charles C Thomas, 1972

The Right Way to Eat, Miriam Polunin, J M Dent/Europa, 1984

Tracking Down Hidden Food Allergies, W G Crook, Professional Books, 1980

The Whole Health Manual, Patrick Holford, Thorsons, 1983

Chapter 2 – Vitamins and Minerals

The Encyclopedia of Food and Nutrition, Jo Rogers, Merehurst, 9 Trinity Centre, Park Farm, Wellingborough NN8 3ZB.

Chapter 3 – Hormones

How Diet can Help Your PMS, Mrs Wendy Holton, Available from NAPS (see address in Appendix)

On the Receiving End, Rev Tom Dalton, Available from NAPS (see address in Appendix)

Once a Month, Dr Katharina Dalton, ISBN 0-00-636658-9

The Pre-menstrual Syndrome and Progesterone Therapy, Dr Katharina Dalton, ISBN 0-433-07092-7

Depression after Childbirth, Dr Katharina Dalton, ISBN 0-19-282228-4

Pre-menstrual Syndrome Illustrated, Dr Katharina Dalton, ISBN 0-946796-41-6

Pre-menstrual Syndrome Goes to Court, Dr Katharina Dalton, ISBN 0-946796-42-4

Pre-menstrual Syndrome – Your Options, Helen Duckworth, Attic Press, ISBN 0946211-671

Chapter 4 – Relaxation

Hatha Yoga, Theos Bernard, Rider

Office Yoga, Julie Friedeberger, Thorsons

Relax and be Happy – Techniques for 5 to 18 Year Olds, Self Care Health Books, Jane Madders

Stress and Relaxation, Macdonald Optima, Jane Madders

Tai Chi for Two: the Practice of Push Hands, Paul Crompton, Shambala

Understanding Stress, The Consumer's Association

Way of Harmony: A Guide to the Soft Martial Arts, Howard Reid, Unwin Hyman

Yoga and the Bhagavad Gita, Tom Macarthyr, Aquarian Press

Yoga Book for Women, P O'Brien, Thorsons

Chapter 6 – Low Blood Sugar

Beat Sugar Craving, Maryon Stewart, Vermillion

Body, Mind and Sugar, Abramson and Pezet, Holt and Rhinehart

Is Low Blood Sugar Making You a Nutritional Cripple? Ruth Adams and Frank Murray, Larchmont Books

Low Blood Sugar (Hypoglycaemia) – The 20th Century Epidemic? Martin L Budd, Thorsons

Muscle Management, Liz Andrews, Thorsons

Sweets Without Sinning, Gwyneth Dover, Sidwick Softbacks

What is Kinesiology? Gordon Dickson, Booklist, 78 Castlewood Drive, Eltham, London SE9

Chapter 7 – Detoxification

A Cancer Therapy, Max Gerson, Gerson Institute

Against All Odds, Dr Hugh Faulkner, Community Health Foundation

The Detox Diet Book, Belinda Grant, Optima

Chapter 8 – Aromatherapy

Aromatherapy, Micheline, ArcierHamlyn

Aromatherapy – An A-Z, Patricia Davis, C W Daniels

Aromatherapy – A guide for home use, Christine Westwood, Kerbina

Aromatherapy for Common Ailments, Shirley Price, Gaia Books

Aromatherapy for Everyone, Robert Tisserand, Penguin

Aromatherapy – Massage with essential oils, Christine Wildwood, Element

Aromatherapy – The encyclopedia of plants and oils and how they may help you, Healing Arts Press

Complete Aromatherapy Handbook – Essential oils for radiant health, Suzanne Fischer-Rizzi, Sterling

The Directory of Essential Oils, Wanda Sellar, C W Daniel Company Ltd

The Encyclopedia of Essential Oils, Julia Lawless, Element Books

The Fragrant Pharmacy, Valerie Ann Worwood, Macmillan

The Joy of Aromatherapy, Cathy Hopkins, Angus and Robertson

Subtle Aromatherapy, Patricia Davis, C W Daniel

Vital Oils, Liz Earle, Ebury Press

Chapter 9 – Homoeopathy

The Barefoot Homoeopath, Madelein Harland and Glen Finn, Hyden House Ltd, Little Hyden Lane, Clanfield, Hampshire, PO8 0RU

Homoeopathy, Dr Ann Clover, Thorsons

Chapter 10 – Herbal Treatment

The Illustrated Herbal Handbook for Everyone, Juliette de Bairacli Levy, Faber and Faber

The New Holistic Herbal, David Hoffman, Element

Chapter 11 – Mind Control and Psychology

Adler's Place in Psychology, Lewis Way

The Awakened Mind: Biofeedback and the Development of Higher States of Awareness, N Coxhead and M Cade, Wildwood House

Basic Applications of Adlerian Psychology, Edith A Dewey

Beyond Biofeedback, E Green and A Green, Knoll

Biofeedback: An Introduction and Guide, D Danskin and M Crow, Mayfield Publishing Co

Gestalt Therapy, F Perls, P Goodman and R Hefferline, R Souvenir Press

Hypnotherapy; A Modern Approach, W Golden et al, Pergamon

Hypnotherapy, is it for you?, R Sleet, Element

Introduction to Psychotherapy, D Brown and J Pedder, RKP

Man Controlled, M Karlins and L M Andrews, Free Press

New Mind, New Body, B Brown, Bantam Books

The Practice and Theory of Individual Psychology, Alfred Adler

Real Health, A Poteliakhoff and M Carruthers, Davis Poynter

The Red Book of Gestalt, by Houston, G Rochester Foundation

The Relaxation Response, H Benson, Fontana

Psychotherapists; A Collection of Basic Writings, R Assagioli, Thorsons

Stress Management, E Charlesworth, Corgi

Stress Reduction, L J Mason, Cel Arts

What We May Be, P Ferruci, Thorsons

You and Autogenic Training, C Rosa, E P Dutton

You Must Relax, E Jacobson, Unwin

Chapter 12 – Bach Flower Remedies

The Bach Flower Remedies – Illustrations and Preparation, Nora Weeks and Victor Bullen

The Bach Flower Remedies Step by Step, Judy Howard, C W Daniel

Bach Flower Therapy, M Scheffer, Thorsons

The Bach Remedies Repertory, F J Wheeler

Dictionary of the Bach Flower Remedies, T W Hyne-Jones

Flower Remedies – Natural Healing with Flower Essences, Christine Wildwood, Health Essentials

Flowers to the Rescue, G Vlamis, Thorsons

Handbook of the Bach Flower Remedies, Philip M Chancellor, C W Daniel

Heal Thyself, Edward Bach, C W Daniel

An Introduction to the Benefits of the Bach Flower Remedies, Jane Evans

The Healing Herbs of Edward Bach, M and J Barnard, The Flower Remedy Programme

The Medical Discoveries of Edward Bach, Physician, Nora Weeks, C W Daniel

The Original Writings of Edward Bach, J Howard and J Ramsell, C W Daniel

Questions and Answers, John Ramsell, Bach Centre

The Story of Mount Vernon, Judy Howard

The Twelve Healers and Other Remedies, Edward Bach

Chapter 13 – Spiritual Healing

Mind Magic, Betty Shine, Bantam Press

Chapter 15 – Acupuncture, Acupressure and Shiatsu

Acupressure for Common Ailments, Chris Jarmey, Gaia Books

Acupuncture and You, Dr Louis Moss, Paul Elek Books

Acupuncture from Ancient Art to Modern Medicine, A Macdonald, Unwin Paperbacks

Acupuncture: The Ancient Chinese Art of Healing, F Mann, Vintage Books

Acupuncture Therapy, M Austin, Thorsons

The Acupuncture Treatment of Pain, L Chaitow, Thorsons

A Beginner's Guide to Shiatsu, Jane Downer, HHodder and Stoughto

The Book of Shiatsu, Paul Lundberg, Gaia Books

First Aid at Your Fingertips, D Lawson-Wood and J Lawson-Wood, C W Daniel

The Foundations of Chinese Medicine, Giovanni Macioci, Churchill Livingstone

The Layman's Guide to Acupuncture, Y Manaka and A Urquart, Weatherhill

Modern Chinese Acupuncture, G T Lewith and N R Lewith, Thorsons

The Natural Healer's Acupressure Handbook, M Blate, Routledge and Kegan

Shiatsu: The Complete Guide, Chris Jarmey and Gabriel Mojay, Thorsons

Shiatsu Workbook: A Beginner's Guide, Nigel Dawes, Piatkus

Thorsons Introductory Guide to Shiatsu, Chris Jarmey, Thorsons

Traditional Acupuncture: The Law of the Five Elements, D M Connelly, Centre for Traditional Acupuncture, Columbia, Maryland USA

Zen Shiatsu, Shizuto Masunaga, Japan Publications

Chapter 16 – Miscellaneous

Moon Madness – And Other Effects of the Full Moon, Paul Katzeff, Hale

Art Therapy

Art as Therapy, T Dalley, RKP

The Inward Journey; Art as Therapy, M Keys, Open Court

Crystal Healing

Crystal Healing, Edmund Harold, The Aquarian Press

The Crystal Heart, Ra Bonewitz ,The Aquarian Press

The Crystal Oracle, LeRoy Montana, Linda Waldron & Kathleen Jonah, The Aquarian Press

The Crystal Workbook, Ursula Markham, The Aquarian Press

Dance Therapy

The Mastery of Movement, R Laban, Northcote House

Personality Assessment Through Movement, Marion North, Northcote Press

Metamorphic Technique

Finding Your Feet, Mary Lambert

The Metamorphic Technique – Principles and Practice, Gaston Saint-Pierre and Debbie Boater Shapiro, Element Books

Metamorphosis – a text book on Pre-Natal Therapy, Robert StJohn

Principles and Practice of the Metamorphic Technique, Gaston Saint-Pierre and Barbara d'Arcy, Thompson

Rebirthing

Rebirthing: The Science of Enjoying All of Your Life, P. Laut, Trinity

Regression Therapy

Other Lives, Other Selves, Dr Roger Woolger, Thorsons

Other

Alcohol and Seizures – Basic Mechanisms and Clinical Concepts

Better Health through Natural Healing – How to get well without drugs or surgery, Ross Trattler ND, DO, Thorsons Publishing Group

Herbs and Aromatherapy, Joannah Metcalfe, Webb and Bower

Kitchen Pharmacy, Rose Elliot & Carlo de Paoli, Chapmans.

Meaning and Medicine, Larry Dossey, Bantam.

Migraine and Epilepsy, Jan de Vries, Mainstream Publishing.

*Natural Healing for Women: Caring for yourself with herbs, homeopathy and essential oils,*Susan Curtis and Romy Fraser, Pandora Press.

A New Viewpoint on Epilepsy Causes and Cures, James C Thomson of the Kingston Clinic Edinburgh, The Incorporated Society of Registered Naturopaths .

Super Health, Dr Mark Payne, Thorsons.

Index

H

Hair, 18, 22, 27

Hay fever, 15

Head injuries, 11

Headaches, 16, 44, 97

Heart, 18

Heavy periods, 17

Hellerwork, 103

Herbs, 79

High blood pressure, 33, 44

Homoeopathy, 71

Hormone treatment, 37

Hypnotherapy, 40

Hypoglycaemia, 47, 97

I

IgE test, 22

Immune system, 34

Immunisations, 11

Insomnia, 44, 93

Insulin, 48, 52

Intelligence, 10

Internal pains, 80

Iridology, 104

Irritability, 29

J

Joints, 18

K

Kelp, 34

Kinesiology, 104

L

Lead, 54

Lecithin, 33, 51

Loss of appetite, 17

Loss of balance, 16

Low blood sugar, 26, 27, 37, 47

M

Magnesium, 30, 38, 51, 58

Management of fits, 83

Manganese, 31, 58

Massage, 40, 66, 93

Measles, 11

Meat, 60

Meditation, 40

Mediumship, 104

Melissa, 66

Menstrual pains, 30, 93

Mental apathy, 32

Mental disturbance., 54

Mercury, 54

Metabolism, 21

Migraine, 16, 44, 93, 97

Minerals, 25

Misaligned vertebrae, 44

Mood swings, 18

Mouth ulcers, 18

Music Therapy, 104

N

Nails, 18

Neck or head injuries, 11

Negative emotions, 87

Nervousness, 44

Neurosis, 11

Nightmares, 16

Nutritional therapist, 26

O

Oligo-Elements, 104

Osteopathy, 43

Other rashes, 19

Ovulation, 37

P

Pancreas, 48

Pancreatic Enzymes, 34

Period, 37

Pesticides, 53

Pins and needles, 16

Pituitary Extract, 34

Polarity Therapy, 105

Pollution, 29

Posture, 43

Potassium, 51

Potassium bromate, 20

Pre-menstrual syndrome, 17, 27, 37

Pregnant, 28, 30, 48, 65

Processed foods, 60

Proteolytic Enzymes, 34

Pulse, 18, 21

R

RAST test, 22

Raw Adrenal, 38, 51

Raw Pancreas, 51

Raw Pituitary tablets, 38

Raw Thymus Concentrate, 34

Reading and comprehension, difficulties, 16

Rebirthing, 105

Regression Therapy, 105

Relaxation Training, 41

Rescue Remedy, 88

Resistance to infection, 34

Restlessness, 16

Rewards and Punishments, 83

Rheumatism, 65

Rosemary, 68

S

Salt, 21

Schizophrenics, 32

Seaweed, 52

Sedative, 80

Selenium, 31, 58

Self-hypnosis, 41

Shiatsu, 96

Skin, 19, 27

Skin rashes, 15

Skull, 44

Sleep, 10

Sleep disorders, 16

Slimming, 30

Smoking, 12

Snoring, 16

Snuffly nose, 18

Sodium aluminium, 20

Sore throats, 19

Spine, 43

Spiritual Healing, 91

Spirulina, 52

Stomach pains, 17

Stress, 11, 15, 25, 28, 39, 43, 47, 51, 84, 97

Stress Management, 41

Sugar, 21, 60

Sugar addiction, 47